MORE TH

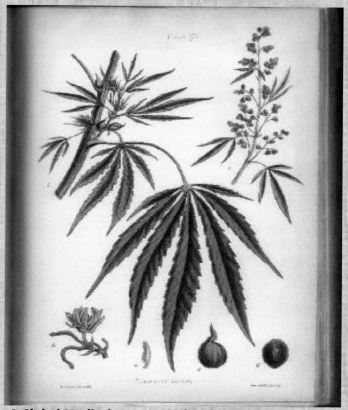

A Global Medical, Economical and Spiritual History of Hemp and *Cannabis*

Olatokunboh M. Obasi M.S

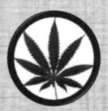

A Global Medical, Economical and Spiritual History of Hemp and *Cannabis*

By Olatokunboh M. Obasi M.S

A Global Medical, Economical and Spiritual History of Hemp and *Cannabis*

This text was reviewed by my teacher and friend Dr. James A. Duke, thank you for your advice and critique. Most importantly, I would like to thank my family and friends who have encouraged and supported me in publishing this wonderful account on a plant that is on the breaking edge of medicinal use in our mainstream healthcare system as well as for supplemental and industrial use. It is amazing the distance it has traveled and the intense, at times, conflicting relationship humans all over the world have had with it. Even though it is currently illicit, it is still a plant with powerful industrial and medicinal value that should be considered legal by the federal government in the future.

Thank you Catherine, Regina and Eric for editing, supporting and critiquing this work!

Nourishing Botanicals, LLC.
www.nourishingbotanicals.com

Nourishing Botanicals LLC. is a registered wellness business of Olatokunboh M. Obasi, M.Sc.

Design and layout: Olatokunboh M. Obasi M.Sc.

This book is intended to be a historical account on the use of marijuana. The compiled data will be useful to physicians, naturopaths, acupuncturists, herbalists, researchers and curious minds. This book is for educational and research purposes only. It is not intended to be a guide nor encourage self medication or use of marijuana as it is still considered illegal.

A Global Medical, Economical and Spiritual History of Hemp and *Cannabis*

This book is dedicated to ALL traditional healers, the shaman of the global villages, my Uncle Arthur Okwemba Bulimo, and my SO very patient children.

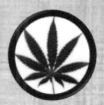

Table of Contents

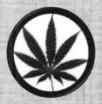

Introduction

"To the agriculturist, Cannabis is a fiber crop; to the physician, it is an enigma; to the user, a euphoria; to the police, a menace; to the trafficker, a source of profitable danger; to the convict or parolee and his family a source of sorrow"
~Mikuriya, 1969 p. 34

Marijuana is an ancient plant cultivated throughout history as far back as 12,000 years. Today, *marijuana* dominates debates in Europe and the United States for its use as a medicine, food and crop. This debate is not new. The purpose of this book is to summarize the global advantages and potential hazards of *marijuana*. It will look through the lens of history using observation, analysis and experience of traditional physicians and healers all over the world. It will provide myths, spiritual and legendary attachments to the plant which spread as rumor throughout the world, thus affecting its image in worlds apart. First I would like to share my personal journey and thoughts in the discovery of *marijuana*. My perspective is global, historical, spiritual and scientific.

At the age of 15, my interest in Bob Marley and the Wailers reggae music and videos of Rastafarian culture was growing. I was mesmerized by reggae music. It was then my interest in *marijuana* became; after all, the stereotype reggae music and *marijuana* are like peas in a pod. I inquisitively questioned about it: What is it? Where did it come from? Why was it smoked? Why is it illegal? As I watched videos of these great musicians smoke in smoke-filled rooms I wondered: is it their relationship with the plant that enabled them to arise to their plane of musical success where many others tried but failed to reach? As I grew older and more interested in Rastafarianism, I had no desire to use *marijuana* because of its bad reputation and I did not want to be associated with its illegal label. I did honor the plant as a sacred symbol of Rastafarianism, as I was at the time impressed with the lifestyle. Years went by and I grew to become an intimate plant lover. I established a non judgmental attitude towards those who chose to smoke *marijuana* around me. As a matter of fact, I came to realize I had grown up and been surrounded by the plant in my native country Kenya many years ago!

Family members and people in the community from Kenya to Tanzania who enjoyed *marijuana* liberally, mostly lived in rural areas. They claimed they could easily become contemplative, be passive and visualize or predict things to come. They claimed it relaxed them and its seed was a nourishing food-source. In my experience, I found that its fragrance was earthy, non addictive and appealing; it always reminded me of burnt White sage, *Salvia apiana* or Mugwort, *Artemisia vulgaris*. In cities like Nairobi, Arusha and Columbus, youthful circles densely created by hip- hop enthusiasts, Rastafarian devotees and college students all held a common interest: seeking freedom by the act of rebellion through the *marijuana* experience. The plant became a symbol of expression for the cause. In some of these circles I had friends who were even involved in the lucrative business of selling *marijuana* which provided well for their families. In contrast, its illicit side was dangerous and scary. I was always afraid for them, whether protecting large sums of untaxed money, police, recreational drugs that could be easily involved in sales, murders and gangs, one had to be prepared for anything usually with weapons. I had heard many stories of people dying or threatened doing the business of *marijuana*.

Politics and law surrounding this plant never made sense to me though. First, it is a plant groomed to grow freely by nature, and humans have found many durable uses for parts of it for eons. From baskets to sails, teas to clothes, it seems to me that it could create an economical profit for many and a nutritious meal from the seed in particular. It grows quickly under harsh conditions and is robust like a weed. Hence, the nickname *Weed*. So why not legalize it for economical gains and nutritious value? Well nowadays

it is legally sold in stores as hemp seed milk, hemp protein
powder, oil or edible seed, at least its nutritious value is
honored. Of course you would have to have some kind of
registration and pay a fee to own a hemp farm. One must
not forget to mention that if green conscious, clothing
stores, many bags and textiles are made from this durable
crop from Silver Spring, Maryland to Johannesburg, South
Africa. However, the fact still remains; to be smoked
without a medical prescription or grown and tinctured, to
make a medicinal tea or herbal remedy is still illegal. Oh
and *please* do not mention that your hemp clothes are
made from *marijuana*. Why? What's the difference
anyway? Keep on reading.

With so many questions, other than those of politics,
economics, medicine, and law of *marijuana* I remain
wondering: what is it about this plant that makes it so
sexy, yet underground, ethereal, mystical, free spirited,
risky, and adventurous? Where are its origins? How long
has it been used? When and where does mankind's
relationship with this plant begin? Is it only Rastafarians
who have always used it, revered it, and held it in a place
of sacredness? Through research I discovered, and decided
to answer these questions in sharing this information with
the public. *Marijuana* has been, is and will be for a while
one of the most provocative and intriguing topics to me.

Now as medical herbalist practitioner, I am even more
curious about its use in botanical medicine. Like most
plants, there is a medicinal side to *marijuana*. *Marijuana's*

7

current attention and use as treatment for modern diseases and conditions, like as an adjuvant to cancer therapy, and analgesic or anti anxiety herb, is becoming very popular and ubiquitous, especially in the West coast of the United States of America. Its media attention is growing, and I predict in less than 5 years from now, it will be a federally legal herb used for wellness as part of mainstream herbal medicine treatment across the USA. Okay, perhaps that's wishful thinking, but not improbable! My belief is that learning *marijuana*'s history is the beginning of knowing this plant and ultimately understanding why people all over the world must have it for medicinal, industrial and other uses. And why some people must avoid it to escape self destruction, crime and illegal behavior. Currently, no matter how many laws are enacted against *marijuana*, people continue to smuggle it, use it and make fortunes and it is important to understand their drive. The journey begins with education. Educating ourselves, our families and our community will lead as to peaceful interactions with a plant so powerful.

First and foremost, we need to look at the roots of *marijuana*. History is the root of all things present; understanding *marijuana*'s history helps us to understand how it has obtained a criminal history label and its potential in the future as medicine and more. Enjoy this brief account as much as I have enjoyed gathering and researching this information.

~in wellness,
Olatokunboh M. Obasi, M.Sc.

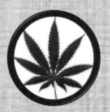

NOMENCLATURE: WHAT'S IN A NAME?

"Look about you. Take hold of the things that are here. Let them talk to you. You learn to talk to them."

~George Washington Carver

Marijuana Family

All plants are ordered by families. *Marijuana's* family formerly *Moraceae*, is currently *Cannabaceae*, the Hemp family which includes over 170 species (United States Department of Agriculture Natural Resources Conservation Service, 2006; Balick & Cox, 1996; Gray, 1894). This family generally has strong antimicrobial and sedating properties. Other family members include *Humulus lupulus* (Hops) an herb used medicinally and recreationally to make beer (Smith, 1883).

Marijuana Botanical Names

Agriculturally it is important to distinguish plants by botanical names in order that one identifies and harvests what is needed correctly. *Cannabis sativa L.* and *Cannabis indica L.* are both botanical names for *marijuana* and were historically used globally. As we will see later, *Cannabis sativa* is found in parts of the world that *Cannabis indica* would later be introduced. One can speculate *C. indica* originated or was introduced by civilizations around the Indus Valley, such as Persia, Caucasus and Northern India (Brown, 1872; Kraemer, 1915). Historically, it appears that people preferred to smoke *Cannabis indica* over *Cannabis sativa* probably because of its stronger psychoactive effects due to its high resinous content (Neill & Smith, 1852; Flora of North America, 2006). The resin contains the psychoactive agents people sought from the plant for recreational and medicinal use (Neill & Smith, 1852).

Marijuana Common Names

There are a plethora of names for this interesting plant, more than I can name in this book. All over the world it was found and named. *Marijuana* was named either after personal association, experience, origin, or after people who popularized it, as we will see in the historical story section of this book. Some of the names for *marijuana* sound familiar and others distant from Western vocabulary. Below I list the most common names used around the world for it. *Marijuana* is the most common known name globally for the plant. The word may have derived from the Mexican-Spanish *mariguana* meaning *Mary and Jane* translated into Spanish as *Maria y Juana* (Bloomquist, 1971). There may also be earlier influence from the Aztec words for the plant *milan-a-huana*. The Portuguese word *mariguango* is very similar to the above variations, it means *intoxicant* (Raman, 2003).

Around the globe *Marijuana* is known as **Hemp, Reefer, Pot, Cannabis**, Mary Jane, and Grass (Naegele, 1980). Bhangaa, Ganjaa, Mang, Charas, **Churrus**, Subjee, Vijayaa, Maadani, Maatulaaní, Trailokya vijayaa, Tribhuvana vijayaa are Ayurvedic/Indian in origin; Qinnab, Ganza, Hashish, Marihuana among Yunani Tibb systems/Indo-Arabian areas; Chancre in France and French speaking regions; **Cannabis** in Scythia (an ancient region which today covers Eastern Europe, Baltic areas and some Persian regions); **Mariguango** in Mexican areas; Dagga in southern Africa, **Umea** by the Xhosa, Matokwane by the Sotho, Nsangu by the Zulu in South Africa, Dachma by the Hottentots of South Africa, Kif in North African regions; Hashish in Syria; Grifa in Spain;

Anascha in Russia; *Kendir* among the Tartar who are descendents of the Mongol people, Momea in Tibet; Konop in Bulgaria; **Konope** in Poland; Kanbun among the people known as the Babylonians presently settled in the Kuwait and Iranian regions; **Dawamesk** in Algeria; *Diamba* or **Maconha** in Brazil; **Bust** or Sheera in Egypt; *Ganjah* in Jamaica; and Huo ma ren, **hu-ma**, ban-ma, *huang-ma* in China, Canamo in Chile and **MALACH** in Turkey (Khare, 2004; Raman, 2003; Van Wyk, 2000; Duke J. A., 1986; Griffith, 1847).

Please Note: Throughout this book, I may use one or any of the above names particularly when discussing the region *marijuana* was used. Otherwise, I will refer to the plant interchangeably as *marijuana* or *Cannabis*. I will distinguish *C. sativa* from *C. indica* to be specific about use and potency where necessary.

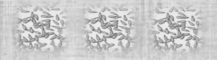

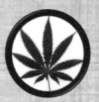

PLANT PARTS USED AND GLOBAL PREPARATION

"Remedy it or welcome it: a wise man's only two choices."

~The Quote Garden

The importance of plant parts, their use and their preparation is the art and science of traditional herbal practice. The whole plant may be considered medicinal however each part may hold different medicinal value. Knowledge of this makes the practice of traditional herbal medicine creative and herbal physicians from ancient societies knew it.

Marijuana Plant Parts

Root

The kind of root *Cannabis* grows is called *taproot* (Naegele, 1980). Around the globe it was dried then used to make powders for a variety of traditional medicinal applications

Stem
The stem is generally what is called *hemp* and is the fiber part of the plant that was used to make textiles, ropes, and paper (Smith, 1883).

Leaves and flowers
In some countries, the leaves and flowers were called *gunjah, ganja, gunza, bhang* or *hashish* (Neill & Smith, 1852). Traditionally, they were used for intoxication, recreation, spiritual, and medicinal purposes. The difference between *ganja* and *bhangaa* must be noted here. *Ganjaa* in India is unfertilized resinous green flowering tops from the female part of the plant and *bhangaa* is dried flower tops as above with leaves or shoots usually mixed with milk (Khare, 2004).

Seeds
All over the world where *Cannabis* has been used, the seeds, also called *hemp* seeds, or *Ma-fen* in China, were used as a nutritious food and oil source (Duke J. A., 1986).
 Hemp seeds are a non-constipating and non narcotic unlike the rest of the plant (Handbook of Ayurvedic Herbal Medicines and Formulae, 2003, Hamilton, 1852). The oil was not only ingested but used as an ingredient for oil paints and varnishes as well (Frank & Rosenthal, 1978).

Resin

Resin is the "blood clot" of the plant. It is this part that many have sought intoxicating pleasure. Resin is obtained by rubbing *marijuana* leaves. In some parts of the world the resin was called *churrus or charas* (Smith, 1883; Griffith, 1847). The resin is a soluble, volatile oil which easily dissolves in alcohol; this active property is also called *cannabin* (Neill & Smith, 1852).

Global Preparations

In the past, people used *Cannabis* for a variety of reasons. Some ingested, smoked or used it medicinally and aroma-therapeutically. The following will give you an idea about the various relationships different regions of the world held with this plant.

Americas

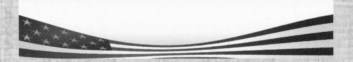

Leaves, flowers and resins were used to make an extract made by boiling dried flowering tops in alcohol until resin was dissolved out and spirit distilled off, then it was rolled up for smoking (called *gunjah*), or macerated to make tinctures (Scudder, 1898). The leaves and flowers were dried and used as an infusion, for cooking and drinking (Naegele, 1980).

India

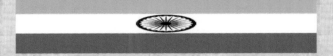

Leaves and stems were macerated in water and made into a
drink mixed with milk called *bhangaa*. Tops of C. *sativa* were
made into *ganjaa*, more potent than *bhangaa* (Smith, 1883).
Ganjaa leaves had been used for baking sweets called *majum* a
combination of milk, ghee, flour and sugar (Touw, 1981). The
most potent *charas*, resin, similar to *hashish* found in Arabia, was
obtained by scraping resin from leaves (Kraemer, 1915). *Charas*
was harvested by naked or leather dressed men passing through
C. *sativa* fields rubbing and crushing against the plants early in
the morning after sunrise, once dew had fallen. The resinous
material was scraped from their bodies then collected for
commerce use (Smith, 1883).

China

The root was ground to a paste to relieve pain from broken
bones and surgical procedures (The Medical Museum: University
of Iowa Health Care, 2006). A salve was made mixing butter, oil
and the ground root to prepare a treatment for burns (The

16

Medical Museum: University of Iowa Health Care, 2006). Khare (2004) tells how Chinese physicians used the flower parts for menstrual disorders and wounds. The achenia considered poisonous, was prescribed for nervous disorders. Seeds and seed oil were recommended as a tonic, demulcent, laxative, antithelmetic, alterative, emmenagogue, to prevent aging, vomiting, poisoning, externally on skin eruptions, wounds, ulcers and applied on the scalp to prevent hair loss (Touw, 1981). Leaves were considered poisonous in Chinese medicine but were carefully freshly juiced then used for gray, falling hair and as a potent antithelmatic remedy (Touw, 1981; Khare, 2004). Lastly, the stalk, bark and root were juiced as a diuretic and to treat gravel in kidneys or gallstones (Khare, 2004).

Africa

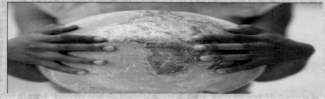

In southern Africa the Hottentots made a drink from the leaves and stems to make a drink like *bhangaa* (Spicer, 2002). The Hottentots also used *dagga* as incense. Here *dagga*[1] was chewed and then smoked out of pipes made from gourds, bamboo stalks and/or coconut bowls (Spicer,2002). In North Africa Muslims

---

[1]*Dagga* should not be confused with *Leonotis nepetifolia* (Wild Dagga) of the Lamiaceae family, a plant applied similarly as *C. sativa* by South, Central and East Africans (Roodt, 1998).

smoked *Cannabis* in glass pipes called *hookahs* (Spicer, 2002). Egyptians too used *Cannabis* as an anti-inflammatory for the uterus and the eyes (Schaffer Library of Drug Policy, 2006).
14th century archeological evidence of smoking bowls in Ethiopia show later use influenced by Arabian fugitives. Congo, Tanzania, and other southern and Islamic nations in Africa, used *Cannabis* during ritual, social and recreational gatherings (Schaffer Library of Drug Policy, 2006).

France

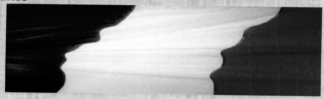

French psychiatrist, Jacques-Joseph Moreau de Tours, practicing at a psychiatry hospital, prepared *Cannabis* green nuggets including, *hashish*, sugar, juice of orange, cinnamon, snail, cardamom, moscada nut, musk, pistachio and pinions. His discovery of *Cannabis* and its use came after a 4 year trip to Egypt and the Middle East (Abel, 1980).

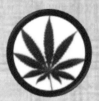

HABITAT ANCESTRY AND ORIGINS

"Native people knew and used various herbs to alter moods, much as we do today, from tobacco to ephedrine, sage, yarrow, morning glory, and various hallucinogenic mushrooms. Some were natural remedies for anxieties and depression, like St. John's Wort. Others were considered the "flesh of the gods," enabling those who ingested them to make spiritual journeys into other realms of knowing and divining information about curing illness."

~from American Indian Healing Arts: Herbs, Rituals, and Remedies for Every Season of Life *by B. Kavasch and K. Baar*

Marijuana Origins

There is substantial speculation that *marijuana* plant ancestry originated in Asia probably on the slopes of the Himalayas or the Altai Mountains to the North (Frank & Rosenthal, 1978). Stone Age trails of *marijuana* cross the Asian continent are obscurely engraved with it, so its exact origin is really unknown. Even though there are several discrepancies about *Cannabis* origination and first use; one

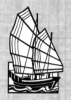 cannot pinpoint it's origination to a single location. However, most primary resources agree with Frank & Rosenthal (1978) that it may have been a native to Neolithic China eventually spread by nomads to Iran, Northern India and the Caucasus regions. As an annual plant found all over the world predominately Northern India, Western Asia and throughout Africa; it is generally cultivated in temperate and warm regions like these (Brown, 1872).

More recently, African *Cannabis* has been shown to yield about 14.06 percent of resin with excellent therapeutic effects; Turkish *Cannabis* contains approximately 9 percent of resin having average therapeutic action (Kraemer, 1915). *Cannabis* prefers to grow in fertile soil, cleared and open to the sun explaining its high resinous yield in Africa. *Cannabis* plants drop seed by the spread of their branches (Griffith, 1847). According to Frank & Rosenthal, 1978, rather than having origins there, the plant was actually *introduced* to the United States. *Marijuana* plants escape or can be cultivated (illegally) throughout the nation except for Alaska. It can be found in well manured, moist farmyards, and in open habitat, waste places, for example, roadsides, railways, vacant lots, in fallow fields and open woods.

Today it is cultivated and used illegally, unless prescribed by a licensed physician or grown with licensure for its fiber, medicine and seed. In the past it was collected in some cases in Mississippi, Iowa and Idaho, but it principally grows in the prairies and plains of central North America (Brown, 1872).

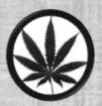

DESCRIPTION FOR *CANNABIS SATIVA*, *CANNABIS INDICA* AND OTHER SPECIES

"The best mind-altering drug is truth."

~Anonymous

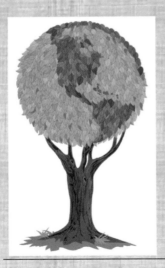

Botany

The following information was summarized from data obtained from several resources the majority being The dispensary of the USA, 25th Ed., 1955, unless otherwise stated. I write this section, like other sections, with great frustration because of the contradictory information among resources. No matter which species we discuss, both

21

marijuana species are basically staminate plants and an annual weed standing from 3-16 ft (Naegele, 1980). Its leaves grow alternate and opposite with a smooth entire point. *Marijuana* petioles range 2-7cm as palmate in appearance with 5-7 lobes that are hairy with 5-7 long leaflets. The leaflets are lance- shaped, toothed or coarsely serrate. Leaf surfaces are whitish green with scattered yellowish brown, resinous dots, stiff with bulbous-based conic hairs. These greenish, sticky, unisexual plants consist of numerous inflorescences. *Marijuana* has staminate flowers with pedicels 0.5-3mm. Its stamens are somewhat

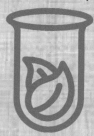 shorter than its sepals and filaments, approximately 0.5-1mm. It consists of pistillate flowers with or without sessiles enclosed by glandular, beaked bracteoles each subtended by a bract as well as a perianth pressed to and surrounding the base of its ovary. The flower or female parts yield the most potent intoxicant odor and substance such as the chief alkaloid THC. THC is a cannabinoid (a type of alkaloid) which stands for delta-9-tetra-hydrocannabinol and is hallucinatory at about 0.3%. The next section will explain it in detail.

Constituents

Marijuana leaves contain over 90 chemical compounds and 60 different types of alkaloids called cannabinoids (Khare, 2004; van Wyk, van Oudtshoorn, & Gericke, 2009). Cannabinoids are important to humans as we produce similar compounds both in effect and structure naturally in

our brain known as endocannabinoids. We have receptors
for these alkaloids for both endogenous and exogenous
purposes. These endocannabinoids are called
anandamides or "bliss molecules" after the Sanskrit word
ananda meaning *bliss* (Iverson, 2000; Van Wyk, 2000).
They affect our nervous system in pain, memory and
inflammation management or shift. In addition to
anandamides, exocannabinoids like that from *Cannabis*
gives us these extra effects to our nervous system.
Therefore, individuals experiencing intolerable pain, for
example, could benefit immensely from *Cannabis* therapy.
Additionally, THCs systemic effects are psychotropic in
nature, the sense that *marijuana* lovers, addicts and
medical practitioners seek, depending on the case (Khare,
2004). THC is solely obtained from female plant resin
produced in *Cannabis sativa* mentions Khare (2004), even
though this is not the same evidence according to Brown
(1872) and Kraemer (1915) who both believe C. *indica* THC is
superior. In general, 15 to 20 percent of the plant contains
cannabin, which is composed of cannabinol. This is a
resinous substance appearing as reddish and oily, but 0.3
percent of cannabin is a yellowish volatile oil consisting of
a sesquiterpene, cannabinene and stearoptene. 1 percent
of the non-flowering plant consists of cannabinene,
volatile alkaloid oil, trimethylamine, and a narcotic with
unpleasant odor in nature (The dispensary of the USA, 25th
Ed., 1955; Kraemer, 1915). THC is insoluble in water,
rendering it difficult to study in *in vivo* and *in vitro* studies
(Iverson, 2000). Seeds of *marijuana* contain 19 percent
protein in the form of oil. Protein can be found in the oil as

enzymes such as lipase, maltase, amylase, urease and tryptase (Touw, 1981).

Species Specific Botany

Cannabis indica: C. *indica* grows 3-4 feet in height and is densely branched, its female part is said to yield more resin than C. *sativa* (Brown, 1872; Kraemer, 1915). This may explain C. *indica* extensive use in drug formulations in the past among Western physicians. The resin contains most of the psychoactive agent, THC (Delta-9-Tetrahyrocannabinol).

Cannabis sativa: Unlike C. *indica*, C. *sativa* can grow as annual up to about 16 feet (The dispensary of the USA, 25th Ed., 1955). Other sources say 6-8 feet (Hamilton, 1852). It grows gangly and loosely branched. In comparison to C. *indica*, its stems are taller, hollow with longer internodes, and less branching. It offers the most productive fiber from its stem, but less superior oil from its seed than C. *indica*. Therefore, its popular application was towards yielding bast fibers and today is used to manufacture hemp fiber for cloths and accessories (Balick & Cox, 1996).

In both species, male flowers are drooping and long, and the female simple and erect. Seeds are small, ash colored and inodorous. Noticeable flowering of these plants were during early summer to fall months in North America. (The above botanical information can be found referenced in the United States Department of Agriculture Natural

Resources Conservation Service 2006 database and The
dispensary of the USA, 25th Ed., 1955).

Marijuana flowering depends on the latitude of its origin.
Plants growing closer to the equator were generally higher
in psycho intoxicants and required a longer induction
period in comparison to those originating further north.
This means that very hot, dry climates produce higher and
richer quantities of resin and not as much fiber (Griffith,
1847). In contrast, mild, humid areas yield less resin but
stronger, durable hemp fiber.   Weaker *Cannabis* plants
have been found in moist conditions as well as where they
closely grow together (Hamilton, 1852).

With that said one can deduce that *C. sativa* may have
originated in northern, cooler, moist climates, and *C.
indica*, in drier hot, tropical climates closer to the equator,
leading to common agreement that *C. indica* is stronger in
THC and other potent constituents. As already writter,
Brown (1872) and Kraemer, (1915) show favorism towards
the Indian Hemp or *Cannabis indica* variety amongst herbal
medical therapists. Herbal physicians as they were called
particularly in North America, had established entrusted
business deals with Indian exporters of the plant in the

past (Frank & Rosenthal, 1978). Yet botanist Dr. Royle[2] stated that not only are both species the same except for the way they are prepared due to climate differences due to where they are grown, but also the robust plant has Persian origins thriving through the coldest winters and the hottest summers (Hamilton, 1852).

Cannabis ruderalis: I was unable to retreive enough substantial information to support all the facets of this species. What I found is that *C. ruderalis* is known to originate in central Asia and produce less THC than *C.sativa* and *C. indica*. It grows much shorter in height and is a less common species of *Cannabis* (Small & Cronquist, 1976).

Sensimella[3]: A seedless version of *Cannabis* whereby the female part of the plant is deprived of pollination from the male plant. The result leads to higher THC or resin exudants. This method of cultivation is credited to the hippies of the 1970's who grew and smoked *Cannabis* culturally within the comfort of their homes (Duckett, 1989).

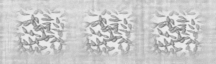

---

[2] A prominent botanist of 1856 Europe who studied *Cannabis*.
[3] A Spanish word meaning *without seed* (Duckett, 1989).

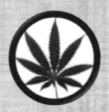

HEMP TRADITONS: GLOBAL MYTH, FOLKLORIC USE AND ORAL HISTORY

"We have to understand our past culture to better understand our present situation. We seem to be in bewilderment of our actions at times without a full understanding of ourselves and the ways of our ancestors' ways that are ingrained into us."

~Credo Mutwa

China

大麻 Chinese historical use of *Cannabis* is extensive and very, very ancient. In the Tung-kuan archives, about 28 A.D, it was recorded that after a war-caused famine, people were encouraged to subsist on wild *Cannabis* and soybeans (Frank & Rosenthal, 1978). An earlier writer of the Han dynasty tells about a record use of the plant as medicine around 28th

century B.C[4] by Emperor Shen-Nung, who "prescribes"
Cannabis for beriberi, constipation, female weakness, gout,
malaria, rheumatism, and absent-mindedness in a book
called the *Pen Tsao Ching* (Bloomquist, 1971; Touw, 1981).
However, some sources reference the Emperor Shen-Nung
as a mythological character of Chinese folk religion, who
was designated as the god creator of agriculture, and a
god mostly worshipped and found in pre-revolutionary
Chinese cosmology (Medical Marijuana ProCon.org, 2006).
Mythological or not, the Chinese, Egyptians and Europeans
used *Cannabis* as prescribed by Shen- Nung well into the
19th century. The Chinese Neolithic culture known as the
Yang-shao, show the earliest evidence of *Cannabis'* flexible
use about 6500 years ago (Frank & Rosenthal, 1978). This
evidence was retrieved along the Yellow River valley by
archeologists.

Persia, Middle East and the Near East

(گ .ش) بوته شاهدانه ، مزد گیاه ، کنف ، بنگ ، حشیش

Persians popularized *hashish,* the name for *marijuana* in
Persia through 12th century A.D. In Arabia the same name
for the plant was used. By 1378, Emir Soudon Sheikhouni
from Joneima, today an Arabian province, attempted to
terminate the use of *hashish.* The etymology of *emir* is
Arabic for *commander, general* or *ruler.* The *emir*
influenced by the government and religious authorities of
that time, claimed that its psychoactive effects were
concerning, probably disrupting manual labor and

---

[4] Some sources say Shen Nung lived earlier, around the 19th century B.C.

economic productivity from workforces (Schaffer Library of Drug Policy, 2006). As a result, he forbade, by law, poor citizens from consuming the plant. Once found growing or in possession, he destroyed the plants and removed the teeth of users before imprisonment. Despite his efforts, consumption persisted and ironically prevailed.

ق نب ,ال ق نب خ يوط ,ذ بات ح ش د يش

As *marijuana* progressed into the Arabian peninsula, tales spread of its ability to grow taller and thicker than flax[5]. In this region, *Cannabis* seeds were burnt as incense called *quannab*[6]. The purpose for *quannab* was to cleanse the mind and make the body proliferate (Spicer, 2002).

India 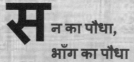 न का पौधा,
भाँग का पौधा

The Hindu revered *Cannabis* as a holy plant. They believed a guardian lives in what they called *bhangaa*[7] (Touw, 1981). "**Bhangaa** is the joy giver, the sky filler, the heavenly guide, the poor man's heaven, the soother of grief... No god or man is as good as the religious drinker of bhangaa" (Medical Marijuana ProCon.org, 2006).

---

[5] Another equally versatile, edible and medicinal plant which grows over 3 feet tall, and commonly used by ancient societies.
[6] Note the word *Cannabis* may have been derived from the root of this word.
[7] Also called *Mang*.

To briefly illustrate the detailed and intricate historical
relationship between *Cannabis* plant and people of India, I
summarized the following from the *History of Marijuana as
Medicine: 2737 B.C to present* (2006):

At Benares, a holy city of the Hindus, and Ujjayini, an
ancient sacred city of the Hindus, students of the
scriptures were given *bhangaa* before they sat to study. In
both cities "yogis took deep draughts of *bhangaa* to center
their thoughts on the Eternal."
Ascetics passed 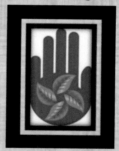 days without food
or drink because of *bhangaa*. Hindu
families abated the miseries of
famine due to this plant. Evidently,
bhangaa helped to curb the pangs
of hunger and thirst for spiritual
practitioners in this region. Aside
from spiritual use, *bhangaa* was
present during ceremonies and celebrations such as
special festivals like weddings. Tradition held the father
responsible to provide *bhangaa* to prevent evil spirits from
accompanying the bride and groom. During other
festivities, *bhangaa* was considered a symbol of hospitality.
Hosts offered their guests a cup of *bhangaa* to avoid being
despised, being considered miserly or misanthropic. In
other parts of this region it was believed that Gautama
Buddha survived by eating only *Cannabis* seeds in the
wilderness (500BC) (Touw, 1981).

30

Mediterranean

Greek, Spanish and Roman physicians and travelers wrote about *Cannabis* after observation and use of the plant. Their knowledge was probably influenced by traders and nomads from Asia and the Middle East. Herodotus[8] a Greek historian called *Cannabis* a Scythian plant (Hamilton, 1852). He wrote about Scythian men who participated in the cult of the dead ritual around 5th century B.C. These men burnt *Cannabis* seeds to create a vapor bath and to induce intoxication during funeral ceremonies (Hamilton, 1852, Schaffer Library of Drug Policy, 2006). Spicer (2002) paraphrases the ritual best, "Small tents into which they placed metal censors containing rocks heated from funeral fires...the Scythians would throw *Cannabis* seeds onto the heated stones to create a thick vapor". 1929 archeologist Professor S.I Rudenko believed Scythian women used *Cannabis* too. Evidence of this was discovered in the 1990's when a female Russian mummy known as both priestess and princess confirmed by a tattoo on her left arm, was found preserved and buried with a container containing *Cannabis* placed next to her (Spicer, 2002). In Rome, around 129-199 A.D, Galen, a prominent physician at the time, promoted the custom of giving guests *hemp* at banquets to bring happiness and

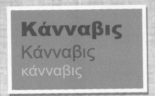

Κάνναβις
Κάνναβις
κάνναβις

---

[8] Known as the world's first historian of the 5th century B.C.

hilarity (Touw, 1981). And then there is the Greek Helen of Telemachus[9] who received *Cannabis* as the "assuager of grief", the Nepenthe[10] of Homer[11], from an Egyptian woman from Thebes (Hamilton, 1852).

Venice

 Marco Polo, the famous Venetian explorer, told tales about the myths of *Cannabis* from his travels to the Middle East. He told stories about a luscious palace belonging to Hasan–al-Sabbah, a wealthy Arabian man, who sent men on assassination missions. Hasan-al-Sabbah was described as the Old Man of the Mountain who bathed in wealth (Schaffer Library of Drug Policy, 2006).

This excerpt from *History of the Intoxicant Use of Marijuana* by Schaffer Library of Drug Policy, 2006 tells what Marco Polo saw:

"Within the territory of the Assassins there were delicious walled gardens in which one can find everything that can satisfy the needs of the body and the caprices of the most exacting

---

[9] Telemachus is the Greek mythological son of Odysseus and Penelope.
[10] Nepenthe was said to originate in Egypt as a medicine for sorrow and forgetfulness. It is mentioned in the fourth book of Homer's Odyssey.
[11] Homer was an ancient Greek poet.

sensuality....Trellises of roses and fragrant vines cover with their foliage pavilion of jade and porcelain furnished with Persian carpets and Grecian embroideries. Delicious drinks in vessels of gold and crystal are served by young boys or girls...the sound of harps mingles with the cooing of doves, the murmur of soft voices blends with the sighing of reeds. All is joy, pleasure, voluptuousness and enchantment. The Grand Master of the Assassins, whenever he discovers a young man resolute enough to belong to his murderous legions...invites the youth to his table and intoxicates him with the plant **hashish**....Here he is informed that he can enjoy perpetually the delights he has just tasted if he will take part in the war of the infidel as commanded by the Prophet".

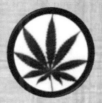

HEMP BUSINESS: GLOBAL RECORDS FOR TRADE AND COMMERCE

"I do not think the measure of a civilization is how tall its buildings of concrete are, but rather how well people have learned to relate to their environment and fellow human beings."

~Sun Bear of the Chippewa tribe

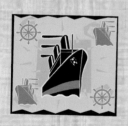 Despite some opinions about the first origination and use of *Cannabis* in China, the earliest records show the beginning of *Cannabis* trade with wandering tribes from ancient peoples such as Aryans, Mongols, and Scythians (Frank & Rosenthal, 1978). They traded *Cannabis* for cotton in India and linen in the Mediterranean. Aryans may have brought *Cannabis* to India as a result of trade and Scythians *Cannabis* to Europe via a northern route. Records also show Greek and Roman

people imported *hemp* fiber from Sicily and Gaul to make ropes and sails. Later apparently, the trade of *Cannabis* grew as it moved from India, west through Persia, Assyria and Arabia about 500 BC (Frank & Rosenthal, 1978). Much later, around 1500 AD[12], busy trade routes between Arabia, North Africa, Turkey, India and Persia formed along the East African coast. Trading avenues allowed Arab traders to eventually introduce *Cannabis* to the southern parts of Africa[13].

Once on the African continent, southern African nomadic San tribe hunters traded *dagga* with the Hottentots in exchange for 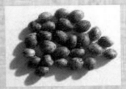 feathers, game, and other products collected from hunting. Meanwhile in Central Africa, business deals were sealed with a puff of smoke from a yard long pipe, resembling that of the Native American tobacco peace pipe, containing *Cannabis* (Frank & Rosenthal, 1978; Spicer, 2002).

---

[12] This date may validate the unsuccessful attempts of Emir Soudon Sheikhouni to terminate the plant in Arabia, his rule was in the 1300s AD when he tried to impose a ban against the use of *Cannabis*.

[13] Confirming the validity of this statement is vague, because some sources say that only *C. indica* must have been introduced to Africa as *C. sativa* was already present and in use there (Schaffer Library of Drug Policy, 2006).

35

Although native peoples of America would disagree, some
sources say that *Cannabis* arrived with slaves and the first
settlers who brought seeds with them (Balick & Cox,
1996). According to David W. Maurer a sociolinguist of the
1940s, *marijuana* was probably introduced to the United
States by way of New Orleans around 1910 with slaves
(Frank & Rosenthal, 1978). Much later during the 19th
century, the American economy grew, and at that time
Cannabis was grown extensively for its fiber and widely
used as medicine (Snyder, 1971). Today, the majority of
hemp in the U.S. is imported from Russia and Italy (Balick &
Cox, 1996).

In a nut shell, *Cannabis'* value as currency was and still is
extremely valuable. *Cannabis* seeds have been used
extensively in trade and travel especially in areas of the
world that held interest in building their economy with
ships and caravans, for instance. No matter where it
landed, it seemed to have been revered as a symbol of
worthy exchange, as it is today. More about its value will
be seen in the next chapter.

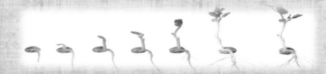

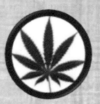

HEMP USE: MEDICAL, SPIRITUAL, COMMERCIAL AND STORYTELLING

"Shaman song, therefore, represents a profound relationship between spirit and matter. The spirit of breath, emerging from within the human organism in the form of song, can be likened to the illumined soul shining through human eyes."

~Joan Halifax, Zen Buddhist, anthropologist, ecologist

Historical Medical Use

Documents and oral traditions about the historical medical use of *marijuana* are found all over the world. *Marijuana* is an herb, a plant that contains medicinal constituents. Historically, cultures around the globe used all parts of the plant and prepared it in various ways for different healing purposes. Most medicinal plants were used in this way because different amounts or types of constituents exist in these parts and therefore applied to specific health needs. The following countries were the most common areas of the world, I found, using *C. indica* or *C. sativa* historically, and applied it traditionally as part of their healthcare system.

Nepal

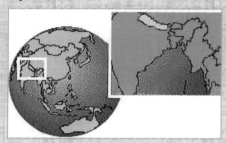

Likely adapted from the Indian Ayurvedic system, Nepali physicians practiced using *C. sativa*[14] or *bhangaa* as medicine. It was traditionally known as an antispasmodic, to relax muscle spasms, as an analgesic, and a sedative (Touw, 1981).

China

Within the writings of Emperor Shen Nung, dated prior to

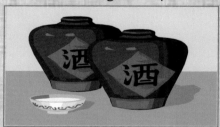

2000 BC, the emperor wrote that *Cannabis* was an important plant applied in treatment for various human illnesses (Frank & Rosenthal, 1978).

---

[14] Notice this resource did not say *C. indica*.

As the 2nd century AD came about, surgeons and physicians
began mixing *Cannabis* with wine to be given to patients
before surgery, as an anesthetic (The Medical Museum:
University of Iowa Health Care, 2006). Hoa-T'o, a Chinese
physician, prescribed *Cannabis* by 200 AD. The herb was
prescribed for malaria, beriberi (a disease caused by a lack
of thiamine or vitamin B1 that affects the nervous system
significantly),   constipation,   rheumatic   pains,
absentmindedness, and female disorders. Furthermore,
the plant was used to alleviate pain, induce sleep, soothe
nervous disorders, and in treatment of eye inflammation
(Touw, 1981).

India

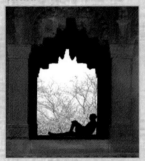

Marijuana was recorded in the
Sutras for religious uses in India.
The Sutras was a religious book
compiled by Sushruta[15] before
1000 BC as an exhilarant (Khare,
2004). The book stated that
marijuana lowered fevers,
promoted sleep, helped in
dysentery, cured sundry illnesses,
stimulated appetite, prolonged
life, quickened the mind, improved judgment, speech
impediments, indigestion, sunstroke, and assisted one to
overcome hunger and thirst (Chaturvedi G.N, 1981; Touw,
1981). In India, *Cannabis* was considered magical. Ayurvedic

---

[15] A legendary ancient Indian physician.

physicians often described *Cannabis* as *vyavayi*. *Vyavayi* is a property of a medicinal plant which assimilates quickly in the whole body surpassing intestinal digestion, therefore leading to quick therapeutic action (Chaturvedi G.N, 1981).

Thailand

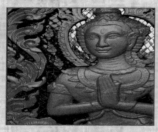 Probably borrowed from India, the healers of Thailand used *Cannabis* to stimulate appetite of the sick, to make them sleep, and to relieve diarrhea or dysentery associated with illness (Spicer, 2002).

Middle East , Arabia and Persia

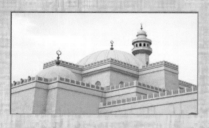 There is immense information showing the medicinal application for *Cannabis* in this region. It was used in Yunani Tibb[16] medicine for numerous ailments, not unlike Chinese and Ayurvedic practitioners (Khare, 2004).

---

[16] Yunani Tibb is an herbal medicinal practice system birthed in this part of the world (Touw, 1981).

Mediterranean

Marijuana was used as a balm for pain before and after childbirth and for disease as stated in 1400 BC documents by Galen[17], the great physician who also recommended the use of *marijuana* in curing gas pains, earaches, toothaches among many other ailments (Hamilton, 1852, Schaffer Library of Drug Policy, 2006).

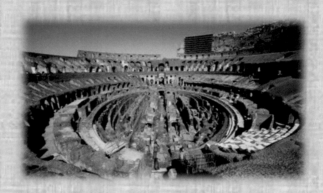

In Greece about 200 BC, there is evidence that *Cannabis* was used as a remedy for earaches, edema and all kinds of inflammatory diseases in Greek medicinal practice (Bloomquist, 1971). Paulus Aegineta[18] juiced the flower tops to relieve pain and obstruction in the ears and used the "fruit" as a carminative for colic and in flatulence

---

[17] A prominent Roman/Greek physician of the 2nd century A.D.
[18] A Greek physician who studied in Egypt and Arabia extensively and wrote a medical encyclopedia.

41

(Hamilton, 1852). During the reign of Roman Emperor Nero, a surgeon, Dioscorides, praised *Cannabis* for its medicinal properties approximately 70 BC (Bloomquist, 1971). Dioscorides[19] used it as a poultice to soothe inflammation and tumors (Hamilton, 1852).

Other Parts of Europe
In the Czech Republic, scientists discovered that a chemical extracted from the *Cannabis* plant contained antibiotic properties against gram negative bacteria (Touw, 1981). And in Ireland, the Irish physician W.B.O O'Shaunessey discovered analgesic and anticonvulsive dyes in *hemp*, 1839 (Bloomquist, 1971).

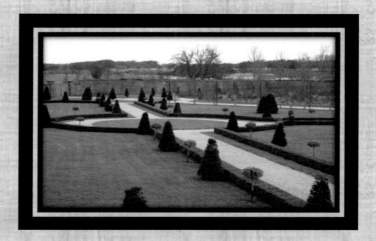

---

[19] Pedanius Dioscorides was a Greek physician, botanist and author of herbal medicine encyclopedias during 40-90 A.D.

United States of America

Physiomedicalists in the U.S used *Cannabis* extensively for medicinal purposes in the 19th century. They applied the plant in treatment of mania, whooping cough, asthma, chronic bronchitis, tetanus, epilepsy and to assist individuals to withdraw from alcohol abuse. Between 1842 and 1890 *marijuana* was the most widely prescribed medicine as a liquid extract (Medical Marijuana ProCon.org, 2006).

Native America

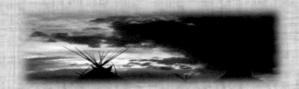

The Iroquois used *C. sativa* to convince patients of recovery from illness, and believed it to be a useful stimulant as well (Moerman, D.E, 1986).

43

Argentina and the Amazon

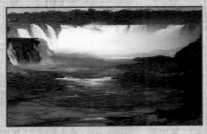 *Cannabis* was considered a panacea herb by healers and herbalists here. It was recommended for tetanus, colic, gastralgia, swelling of the liver, gonorrhea, sterility, impotency, abortion, tuberculosis of the lungs, and asthma (Spicer, 2002). Its root bark was pulverized or decocted to be used as a febrifuge, a tonic, in treatment of dysentery and gastralgia. The ground root was also applied topically to relieve pain. Oil from seeds was extracted to be used in treatment of cancer (Medical Marijuana ProCon.org, 2006). Within the Amazon areas, *marijuana* was cultivated to be used as a hallucinogen and narcotic (Duke & Vasquez, 1994).

Persia, Arabia and the Middle East
Ibn Sina[20] and Yahya ibn Sarafyun[21] both recommended *Cannabis* as a harmless aphrodisiac and said it to be a barely addictive plant, unlike opium. A drink called *Bengi*

---

[20] Known in Europe as Avicenna, a great Persian physician and metaphysician of 10-11th century A.D.

[21] Known in Europe as Serapion, a Syrian Christian physician of 9th century A.D.

or *Kidibengi* made with *Cannabis* was used to release exhaustion and enhance sexual desire (Hamilton, 1852).

Africa

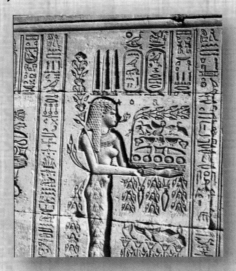

Cannabis is not indigenous to the sub-Saharan African continent, it is speculated that it arrived with Arab/Islamic traders (van Wyk, van Oudtshoorn, & Gericke, 2009). If true, like all indigenous people, Africans learned how to apply the plant for religious, medicinal and recreational purposes over 6 centuries ago when *Cannabis* arrived there through trading routes (Spicer, 2002). *Cannabis* was used on the continent to restore appetite, relieve pain of hemorrhoids, as an antiseptic and in treatment of sore eyes.   The Hottentots in the southern part of Africa, were applying *Cannabis* to snake bites, to facilitate childbirth by the Sotho; and in Rhodesia[22], for anthrax, malaria, black water fever, blood poisoning, dysentery, and as an asthma remedy (van Wyk, van Oudtshoorn, & Gericke, 2009; Schaffer Library of Drug Policy, 2006). In a 2000 BC[23] Egyptian document, there tells of *Cannabis* used for "cooling the uterus", this could mean any female uterine disorders such as dysmenorrhea, fibroids, and infertility (Abel, 1980).

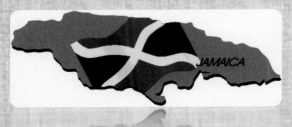

Jamaica
Cannabis was well used as a medicine in Jamaica. Healers claimed *Cannabis* to be used to treat upper respiratory infections, asthma, intestinal problems, glaucoma, gonorrhea, wasting diseases due to malnutrition, infant

---

[22] The colonial name for the southern African country today known as Zimbabwe.
[23] Notice how old this date is, yet some texts still speak of *Cannabis* as a recently introduced plant on the continent of Africa. This date is as old as some of the Chinese writers and physicians who were using the plant at that time and maybe there is confusion between *C. sativa and C. indica*. *C. sativa* might have already been on the continent.

diarrhea, endemic fevers, teething, and for skin burns and abrasions (Schaffer Library of Drug Policy, 2006).

Historical Spiritual Use

Spiritual practices varied all over the world. *Cannabis* bridged a strong relationship between healing and spirituality in many societies. Spirituality was seen as a powerful mystical transformation, a phenomenal disposition and a sacred place within one's body, time and space. *Cannabis* was revered as a plant that could take the individual into elevated levels of consciousness. It was desirable to get there. Sexual feelings were very much a sensation sought for during spiritual elevations especially in Asia. *Cannabis* was a great tool during this sojourner. The reason for sexual attainment during spiritual elevation is unclear to me, except for the fact that the experience of the sense of orgasm may have been perceived as similar to the sense of spiritual bliss. Death too was seen as a spiritual passage in many cultures. *Cannabis* played a symbolic role in burials and beliefs accompanying the deceased as they found their way through the afterlife.

Middle East, Persia

Cannabis was already popular within this area prior to Islam. Once Islam arrived during the forbiddance of alcohol, *Cannabis* became a substitute to followers of the religion (Schaffer Library of Drug Policy, 2006).

Nepal
On feast days, *Cannabis* was distributed at the temples of all Shiva followers (Touw, 1981).

Mediterranean and Other Parts of Europe
Democritus, the laughing philosopher, spoke of *Cannabis* as a drink to be combined with myrrh and wine to enhance visions (Touw, 1981). In the Old Testament Aramaic translation of the Bible, *Cannabis* was recorded as an incense and intoxicant. In the same text there is mention of holy oil. Channeled by Moses from God, a holy oil used in healing contained myrrh, sweet cinnamon, *keneb bosom* and cassia; *keneb bosom* is literally sweet reed and speculated to be synonymous to *Cannabis* (Touw, 1981; Spicer, 2002).

China

In *the Pên-ts'ao Ching*[24], *marijuana* is addressed as having a

potent influence on the psyche (Khare, 2004). The book tells of both *Cannabis* medicinal and spiritual use in practice in China. The pharmacopoeia mentions that if *marijuana* fruits (flowering tops) were taken in excess they made one 'see devils', which is translated as hallucinations (Frank & Rosenthal, 1978; Spicer, 2002). In addition, if taken for a long period of time, it can cause one to communicate with spirits and decreases heaviness in one's body. Shamans used *Cannabis* stalks as "a symbol of power to drive away evil" (Spicer, 2002). To obtain immorality, Taoists of the 1st century burnt *Cannabis* seeds as a hallucinatory (Touw, 1981). In Touw (1981) article further states a Taoist priest of the 5th century A.D who comments on the *Pen Ts'ao Ching* in his own writings *Ming-I Pieh Lu* that, "*Cannabis* is used by necromancers, in combination with ginseng to set forward time in order to reveal future events". In death rituals, *Cannabis* seeds were burnt on metallic tripod censers and used during funeral rites to bring about trances, much like the Scythians.

India

Aryan religions introduced *marijuana* to India, thereafter *marijuana* became a sacred plant in the practice of

---

[24] The oldest pharmacopoeia in China, about 3000 years old (Khare, 2004).

Hinduism (Schaffer Library of Drug Policy, 2006). According to Indian mythology, *bhangaa* was a gift from the gods, "*bhangaa's* spirit was worshipped to free distress and relieves anxiety", recorded in the *Atharva Veda* from the four Vedas (Frank & Rosenthal, 1978).

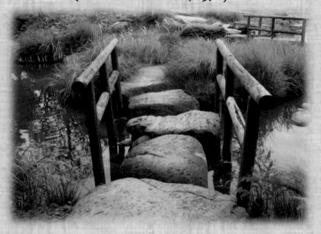

Smoked *Cannabis* was used to enhance concentration in prayer in order to prevent distractions from worldly things and to concentrate on the Supreme Being. The Hindus considered *Cannabis* as the heavenly guide; the soother of grief (Touw, 1981). In addition, the *Atharva Vedas* tell of five sacred plants where a guardian angel resides within their leaves, *Cannabis* being one of them. The use of *Cannabis* was to be applied as protection against spiritual and physical enemies.

The Indian god Shiva was called the Lord of *bhangaa* (Spicer, 2002; Touw, 1981). Shiva was also known as the god of sex in India, hence *bhangaa's* popular association to Tantric religious yoga sex, historically. Prior to the yoga ritual, a bowl of *bhangaa* would be placed before the participant; he[25] would recite a mantra to the goddess Kali[26] and then drink the *bhangaa* potion. The goal of the Tantra was to initiate the unification of the body, mind and spirit through yoga and continuous sexual episodes. *Bhangaa's* role in this act was to optimize the experience. Elsewhere, Hindu mystics smoked *charas* in prayer ceremony called *Puja*. Holy men believed that *charas* brought them closer to their gods (Touw, 1981).

Tibet
Before enlightenment Gautama Buddha ingested one *hemp* seed daily. Until today, depictions of his begging bowl commonly have the serrated leaves of *Cannabis*. *Cannabis* was considered a sacred plant in Tibet. *Cannabis* was used in meditative ritual ceremonies by the Mahayana Buddhists which could have possibly been used to attain sexual highs as well (Touw, 1981).

Brazil
In Brazil, *Cannabis* was used to cure the sick. It is said that African Angolan slaves and their descendents performed spiritual practices involving *Cannabis*. These influenced

---

[25] Usually men participated in the rituals.
[26] *Kali* is a goddess entity in Hinduism who gives Shiva power and energy.

51

Catimbo Indian spiritual practices as well, to use *marijuana* in the purpose of inducing divination, revelation of secrets, and mystic hallucinations (Schaffer Library of Drug Policy, 2006).

Jamaica

It is common knowledge that Rastafarians[27] used, and continue to use, *ganjah* as a politico-religious lifestyle; it is considered the "holy herb" (Spicer, 2002). It was believed that when inhaled it allowed the Rastafarian to be a free Black person. The herb was used as the key to unlock understanding of self, universe, and God. Its role was to take one to cosmic consciousness, to permit one to arrive to the level of reality which allows for fusion between people and all living beings; an existence not ordinarily perceived by non Rastafarians. The smoking of *ganjah* was seen as rites of passage from adolescence to adulthood (Spicer, 2002). Smoking with others symbolized camaraderie, equality, belonging, a sign of friendship and trustworthiness.

---

[27] The most popular global religious culture, that heavily believes in the daily use of *Cannabis*. This religion arose from this region as Africans fled slavery in body and mind in the New World.

Africa

This source claims that Cannabis was already found in the
Zambezi Valley before
Islamic missionaries
popularized it to the
continent (Frank &
Rosenthal, 1978).

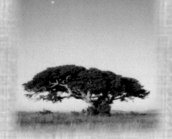

Historically, tribes from
Congo, East Africa, around
Lake Victoria and South
Africa all smoked, and still
smoke *marijuana* in ritual and
leisurely settings. *Cannabis*
was seen as the sacramental
right of all humans.

The ancient Riamba people of the Congo believed
marijuana was provided by a god whose purpose was to be
protector of physical and spiritual harm (Frank &
Rosenthal, 1978). As a result, Riamba warriors used it
ritually in preparation for battle (Schaffer Library of Drug
Policy, 2006).

East of Congo, the Baluba tribe, now found in Tanzania,
had used *Cannabis* for feasts and state observances as well
as a leisurely evening pastime (Schaffer Library of Drug
Policy, 2006). The Ethiopian Zion Coptic Church believed
marijuana was the godly creation given in the beginning of
the world (Spicer, 2002). Its purpose was to be used as a
fiery sacrifice to their Redeemer during obligations.

Turning to the Zulu of South Africa, like the Congolese,
they believed that *dagga* strengthened the spirit prior to
the onslaught at battle (Schaffer Library of Drug Policy,
2006).

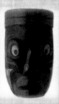

Native America
Contrary to Western consensus that *Cannabis* was
introduced to the Americas via slavery or European
influence, there is some oral evidence of its use here many
years prior to their arrival. Ancestors of Native Americans
of the north were said to have smoked *Cannabis*. Some
elders were known to smoke the flower tops in rolled corn
paper called a "joint" as a daily ritual to give thanks to
Great Mother (Spicer, 2002).

In Central America, Mexican Indians are said to have
practiced a communal curing ceremony using *Cannabis* in
worship as a plant representing the heart of God and an
earth deity. The plant used in the ceremony as a
sacramental gift, *Cannabis*, was known as Santa Rosa
(Spicer, 2002).

Historical Commercial Use

Everywhere in the ancient world the use of natural fibers to create everyday items was found. Flax, sisal, cotton and *Cannabis* made this possible. According to Balick & Cox (1996) as early as 8000 BC[28] there is evidence that baskets, paper, clothing, shoes, and ropes are examples of the types of ubiquitous things that were made from the fibers of *Cannabis* or *hemp*. Until 1883, *Cannabis* was used in the manufacturing of paper for Gutenberg Bibles and King James Version Bibles. More stunningly, drafts of the U.S Declaration of Independence were also made by this plants fiber. It was known to be a robust and versatile material and its global primetime lasted from the 13th century B.C to mid 19th century A.D to make strong, long-lasting ship sails (Balick & Cox, 1996).

Today, we rarely find any of these items made from *Cannabis* anymore. Only recently they are slowly being reintroduced into mainstream society as clothing items and accessories.

---

[28] Note this is an earlier date than any medicinal record used in this book.

China

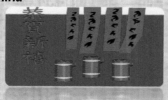 During the 5th century BC, *Cannabis* fiber was used for ship sails and as a major paper fiber up until 1883. *Hemp* fibers were woven into fabric as far back as 5000[29] years. According to Balick & Cox, 1996, hemp garments were finely woven and used in the burials of the Chinese celebrities of the time from the Western Han dynasty ruling (260 B.C. – A.D 24). Bast fibers of male plants were used to weave cloth used for most Chinese garments and Tang dynasty shoes ruling (A.D 618 – 907). *Hemp* paper was obtained from old *hemp* rags and fish nets. It was recycled into a durable kind of paper a couple centuries before the claimed invention by Ts'ai Lun. Some of this paper has currently been retrieved at grave sites near Xi'an of the Shaanxi province of Emperor Wu of the Han Dynasty predating 180 BC (Frank & Rosenthal, 1978; Balick & Cox, 1996; Touw, 1981).

In their discussion, Frank & Rosenthal (1978) show evidence of *Cannabis* use along the Yellow River valley where the Yang-shao culture flourished. This evidence is written in the early classics of the Chou dynasty. The Yang-shao used *hemp* fiber for clothing, fishing nets, hunting nets, and ropes 6,500 years ago. Records show the culture

---

[29] This date confirms that *Cannabis* may have first been used for its fiber prior to discovery for its medicine (Hamilton, 1852).

had no written language but instead communicated by tying knots in ropes made from *hemp*.

As already mentioned above, in 1st to 2nd century BC, the use of the whole plant of *Cannabis* in China was already prevalent. Sought for its fiber source; seed considered one of the five sustainable grains; the others were rice, millet, barley and soybeans[30]. Eventually as technological advances developed in China, the ancient Chinese learned to extract oil from the seeds by pressing (Frank & Rosenthal, 1978). The oil was valuable in that 20 percent oil was yielded by weight. After pressing, the residue still yielded 10 percent oil and about 30 percent protein. Consequently, the oil was used for cooking, fuel lamps, lubrication, and base in paint, varnish, and soap making. The protein was compacted to make *hemp* cakes which were used as animal feed (Frank & Rosenthal, 1978).

Tibet
Tibetan monks were impressed by the quality of paper coming from China. They probably requested for *hemp* paper, as monastic histories are recorded on hemp paper (Touw, 1981).

Africa

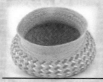 *Kif* was used in North Africa for architectural purposes. *Kif* rooms were formed for family and group gatherings for song, dance and storytelling

---

[30] Although a bean, it was considered a staple and sustainable crop.

(Schaffer Library of Drug Policy, 2006). Among the Tswana of Botswana, *dagga* was used to make cordage and clothing (Schaffer Library of Drug Policy, 2006).

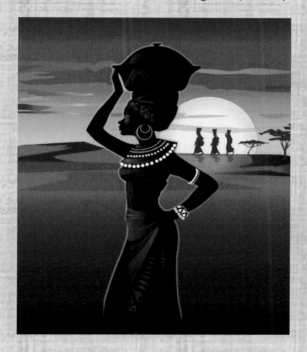

Historical Stories and Use
Persia, Assyria, Arabia
By 500 A.D. *marijuana* spread with the dispersion of Islam as *hashish*, reaching far places such as Africa (Frank & Rosenthal, 1978). Schaffer Library of Drug Policy (2006)

shares an intriguing tale describing the relationship between assassins and *marijuana*. I retell it here.

During the 11th century AD, a man named Al-Hasan ibn al-Sabbah, the same man Marco Polo told stories about, established an enclave overlooking a strategic caravan route near Baghdad. By 1090, he stopped attending his Muslim teachings of the day and founded a sect of practitioners called the *hashishin* after his name *al- Hasan*. As a result of robbing caravans on the road to Baghdad this sect became rich building luscious palaces and gardens for their followers. As time went by, the *hashishin* numbered over 12,000 attracting many young men into the cult receiving their education in the arts of robbery and assassination. Travelers to the court of al-Hasan described it as an earthly paradise, where young men were sedated by a beverage derived from *Cannabis*, and lived in bliss to satisfy their needs. Al-Hasan employed many men to spread his religion and ideologies and killed anyone who opposed of them. The reward for the *hashishin* was their promise to eternity in paradise where they would live as they did in al-Hasan's palace. His soldiers known as *assassin*[31] were fierce, determined, and extraordinarily successful. Their use of *Cannabis* predates the 11th century in Persia.

---

[31] A modification of the word *hashishin*.

Europe

After Napoleon's Egypt campaign in the 1800s his troops returned to France with a new habit; consumption of *Cannabis* resin, *charas* or *hashish* (Schaffer Library of Drug Policy, 2006). Initially, it was used in the treatment of mental illness, then later its use changed from therapy to recreation in Paris. *Le Club des Haschischins* was a recreational group formed as a result of the popularity of *Cannabis* and the enjoyment of sharing each other's "visions". These kinds of meetings were held at the Hotel Pinodan on the Ile Saint-Louis around 1844 (Schaffer Library of Drug Policy, 2006).

In various parts of Europe *Cannabis* was cultivated to manufacture rope particularly in Rome and Greece (Griffith, 1847). Evidence of *Cannabis* through pollen analysis, was found in Norway dating 400 B.C, Sweden 150 A.D and Germany and England 400 A.D (Frank & Rosenthal, 1978).

Middle East

In the ancient Middle East near Jerusalem, archeologists discovered *Cannabis* in the abdominal cavity of a young woman who died of child birth during the 4th century BC. It was concluded that the "drug" was used as an inhalant to reduce pain and increase uterine contractions. Unfortunately, cause of death was not specified as reported in the Medical Marijuana ProCon.org (2006).

Brazil

Spicer (2002) tells how Angolan slaves from the southwest
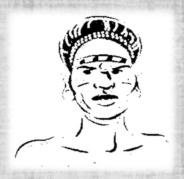
coast of Africa brought *Cannabis* as they worked on the plantations of northeastern Brazil. They carried the seeds tied in cloth dolls, then attached it to their clothing. Slaves planted these seeds while working on the plantation. In 1817, Dona (Queen) Carlota Joaquin, a slave owner, was dying from an anonymous illness. She asked her favorite Angolan slave to make an infusion of *diamba do Amazonas* or *Cannabis* and arsenic, and administer it to her.

Dona Carlota slipped into a numbing euphoria while dying as the potent *diamba* analgesic properties eased her pain.

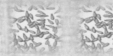

HEMP HEALING: PHYSIOLOGICAL ACTIONS AND SPECIFIC INDICATIONS

"The art of healing comes from nature, not from the physician. Therefore the physician must start from nature, with an open mind."

~Philipus Aureolus Paracelsus 1493-1541, physician, botanist, occultist

Physiological action is a technical term commonly used by medical practitioners, in this case the medical herbalist, to describe the way herbal properties act on the physical body. After an herb is ingested and digested, our bodies breakdown chemicals in the herb. There are several chemicals each herb consists of and they are released throughout our bodies to become medicinally beneficial. This section discusses what and how *Cannabis* treated the physical body after ingesting it as a tea, powder, tincture or extract. Traditional practitioners observed, identified and assessed their patients' illnesses to determine

whether *Cannabis* would be a useful remedy or not. This is
exactly what the term *specific indication* means.

Physiological Actions

China

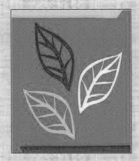
Used in China as an analgesic during
surgical procedures, as a laxative,
alterative, emmenagogue, blood
purifier, antidepressant, anti-malarial,
anti-diarrheal and to enhance
appetite. Topically used also as an
anodyne, and in treatment of burns.
The above information was obtained
from the Medical Museum: University
of Iowa Health Care, 2006.

India

Indian physicians used *Cannabis* for anesthetic purposes,
additionally as an anti-phlegmatic (to move excess mucous
out of the body accumulated in the eyes as intraocular
congestion, the nasal passage or other parts of the body
as tumors), appetite stimulant and as a hypnotic in the
form of *bhangaa* as mentioned in the *Sushruta Samhita*[32]
(Bloomquist, 1971; Touw, 1981). For the healthy population
it was recommended as an aphrodisiac and as a general
health rejuvenator (Handbook of Ayurvedic Herbal
Medicines and Formulae, 2003).

---

[32] An early record of medical works dated 400 B.C-600 A.D.

United States
The United States medical herbalists used *Cannabis* as a narcotic, antibiotic (against gram positive bacteria) as in Europe, anodyne, antispasmodic, sedative, aphrodisiac, nerve tonic, urinary tonic and appetite stimulant (Naegele, 1980; Neill & Smith, 1852). They also found the herb very useful as a psychotherapeutic in altering mood and perception, muscle relaxant and anticonvulsant (Snyder, 1971).

Europe
There was little difference in the manner in which *Cannabis* was applied medicinally in Europe to United States. It had a particular reputation as a tonic for immune deficiencies.

Africa
On a continent filled with venomous creatures and persistent critters, *Cannabis* served as a true antiseptic, hypnotic, anodyne, antidote to snake bites, respiratory conditions, antipyretic, uterine sedative and as an eye wash (Schaffer Library of Drug Policy, 2006).

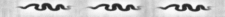

Specific Indications

North America
This area of the continent recorded historical literature
showing *Cannabis* was indicated for the following:
- Burning in the urethra and throughout the urinary
  tract system (Scudder, 1898),
- Frequent micturition with associated burning
  (Scudder, 1898),
- Excitement of men's reproductive function with
  erections, lustful thoughts both conscious and
  unconsciously (Scudder, 1898),
- For neuralgia and other neurological conditions
  such as muscle spasms, sciatica, chronic
  rheumatism, convulsions, sleeplessness, coughs,
  asthma and pertussis (Naegele, 1980, Scudder,
  1898),
- Scudder 1898 further states that it mitigates
  urgent symptoms and is greatly used in treatment
  of gonorrhea, in the "wrongs of the reproductive
  functions" for both men and women,
- Diseases of the bladder and prostate gland, also
  useful for women with hyperesthesia (increased
  sensitivity) of the genitals,
- Also, useful for intraocular pressure from
  glaucoma, multiple sclerosis and nausea of
  chemotherapy (Duke & Vasquez, 1994, Balick &
  Cox, 1996).

Africa
Pre 1700 in various parts of Africa, *Cannabis* was used:
- To treat tetanus,
- Hydrophobia,
- Delirium tremens,
- Infantile convulsions, rheumatism, and other neurological disorders,
- Cholera,
- Menorrhagia,
- Allergies and allergic related conditions like hay fever, asthma, dermatitis, skin diseases and protracted labor during childbirth,
- It was also applied to restore appetite, and relieve pain of hemorrhoids.

Europe
During the medieval era physicians used *Cannabis* in similar ways as North Americans and Africans. It was not until the 1840's that *Cannabis* was studied *extensively* under physicians such as Dr. O'Shaughnessy, Aubert-Roche and Moreau de Tours (Abel, 1980). They and others before them used the plant in the following ways as reported in a 1621 UK medical literature document (Neill & Smith, 1852, Griffith, 1847):

- To induce sleep,
- As a painkiller,
- To soothe nervous disorders,
- To relieve congestion,

- To treat gout and rheumatism
- Malaria,
- Beriberi,
- To treat burns,
- To ease menstrual pain,
- In treatment of depression,
- Treatment for tetanus,
- Hydrophobia,
- Cholera,
- Cataracta lenticularis,
- Relaxation of spasms,
- Well used for gonorrhea.

India
In the Handbook of Ayurvedic Herbal Medicines and Formulae (2003), *Cannabis* was commonly used by the Ayurvedic physician in the treatment of these and 32 other illnesses:

- *Grahani* (chronic colitis, irritable bowel syndrome),
- *Bandhyatva* (male and female sterility),
- *Napumsakatva* (impotency),
- *Atisara* (diarrohea),
- *Ajirna* (indigestion),
- *Apasmara* (epilepsy),
- *Unmada* (insanity),
- *Sula* (colic pain) are just some of the major ones,
- Leprosy,
- Antidote to venomous bites by fish and scorpions,
- As an antipsycotic,

- For all neurological conditions
- Antidiabetic.

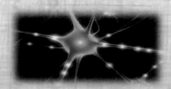 Today, Western research shows *Cannabis* is promising in the treatment of nausea caused by chemotherapy, to fight cancer, and to combat AIDS cases while patients undergo therapy (Khare, 2004). Additional accepted recommendations include abnormal eye pressure caused by glaucoma, arthritis, child birth pain, and for blood pressure in the reduction of essential hypertension (University of Washington, 2006).

Veterinary/Animal Use: THC has been seen as an anticonvulsive reducing these symptoms in cat and rat studies (Khare, 2004). Hemp seeds were used as feed for caged birds (Smith, 1883). For roaming chickens, *Cannabis* was given to fatten, but ancients warned that excessive ingestion would lead to infertility (Hamilton, 1852). East Asian, mainly Chinese, fishermen used *Cannabis* as a fish tranquillzer. Conversley in India, it was used to energize bulls against  amotivational syndrome (Touw, 1981). In Africa, one commonly finds *Acherontia atropos,* Death's Head Hawk Moth, prolific on the continent, feeding on *C. sativa* (Roodt, 1998).

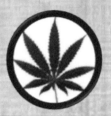

INGESTING HEMP: ENERGETICS, DOSAGE, AND GLOBAL FORMULARY

"To everything there is a season, and a time to every purpose under the heaven; a time to be born, and a time to die; a time to plant, and a time to pluck that which is planted."

~Ecclesiastes 3, Bible

Like many medical herbalists today in the U.S or Europe, traditional practitioners around the world have connected with herbs to treat illnesses. To affirm this intimate connection, it was important to understand every aspect of the plant as a medicine. This understanding was achieved by a refined relationship that had to be established between plant and human being. It began with personal experience and testimony. Careful attention to taste, dose and preparation was needed in order that the medicinal plant was used correctly. Many times discovery of medicinal capabilities began between the practitioner and plant, observing animals, and establishing a plant relationship. The relationship included tasting it, using it to treat one self and others, observing its complex physical form or its simple nature. This relationship, seemingly, could be on two extremes: subjective and objective. Thus, herbalists' opinions could vary about the medicinal effect of each plant. Certainly, to bring forth the healing process, the herbalist treating the individual was sure to develop an intimate relationship with the plant and the patient. The same is true for most herbal and traditional practitioners today. So, *energetics* stands for the energy exuding from the plant and its compatibility with the being experienced through various ways. Sound, color, feeling, taste and odor are some examples.

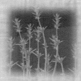

Marijuana Energetics, Taste and Odor:
Its odor is distinctly aromatic, peculiar and narcotic; its taste slightly acrid (Gray, 1894, Kraemer, 1915) also noted as hot (Khare, 2004). The female part of the plant has been said to be bitter and pungent (Handbook of Ayurvedic Herbal Medicines and Formulae, 2003). It is considered a *yin herb* in old Chinese texts that "moisturizes fire", while Perisans via Yunani Tibb, have a rather complex deduction for *Cannabis'* energetics. Other than being a mover of bile, it's initial effects are uplifting, increasing

sexual desire, appetite and excitement. On the contrary, its final effects are melancholic, impotency, edema causing, and creating a disposition for indigestion. In Ayurveda it would be considered a *pittala* herb synonmous to *choleric* in which the Europeans considered it to be according to the four humor system popularized by Galen (Touw, 1981).

Traditional Dosage Europe and United States:
300 to 480 micrograms per kilogram of body weight for ingesting as tea, and 200 to 250 micrograms per kilogram of body weight for smoking therapy (Naegele, 1980). Usually one to five drops of the extract were recommended to add to water or given in teaspoonful doses every two to four hours depending on acuteness of disease (Scudder, 1898).

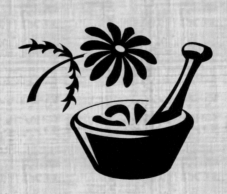

Official Preparations

Medieval Europe

A standard painkiller was prepared with the root for menstrual cramps. Homeopathic tinctures made with male and female flowering tops for headaches, vertigo, hysteria, constipation, nephritis, cystitis, gonorrhea, amenorrhea, infantile leucorrhea and affections of the male sexual organs (Khare, 2004, Abel, 1980). *Hemp* water was seen to be optimal homeopathically for headaches caused by heat and yet causing headaches for those who handled it (Hamilton, 1852).

Dr. O'Shaughnessy[33] treated his patients for rheumatism; cholera and tetanus etc. (See more in the physiological actions and specific indications sections of this book). His personal clinical treatment of tetanus included a tincture of the resinous extract of *Cannabis*, in which he observed immediate relaxation (Hamilton, 1852). Generally, he used *Cannabis* herb, dosed at 1 grain (equivalent to approximately 65mg) with the extract and/or tincture gradually increasing dose from 5-10 drops as needed (Griffith, 1847).

A common preparation was to express juice from the flowering tops of *Cannabis* and add equal amounts of alcohol to it (Hamilton, 1852).

---

[33] An Irish physician of the 1800's who studied in India where he learned folk medicine . He is credited for introducing *Cannabis* to the Western world.

India

Official preparation of *Cannabis* liquid extract or tincture from root or leaf was listed in the 1954 and 1966 Pharmacopeias of India explaining how it was made in detail. *"... the extract was made by boiling the dried flowering tops (ganjaa) in alcohol until the resin was dissolved out and then the spirit was distilled off. The tincture was made by dissolving 64.8 mg of the extract in 3.7 ml of diluted alcohol"* (Neill & Smith, 1852).

In the *Sarngadhara Samhita*[34] *Cannabis* was popularly used in the treatment of diarrhea and as an aphrodisiac. Chaturvedi G.N, (1981) provides a formula, *Jatiphaladi Powder*, prepared by including *Cannabis* for treating several conditions already discussed above:

---

[34] Another Ayurvedic text on medicinal herbs.

Sanskrit Name	Latin Name	Part
Jatiphala	Myristica fragrans	1
Lavanga	Caryophyllus aromaticus	"
Elaci	Elettaria cardamomum	"
Tejpatra	Cinnamomum tamala	"
Dalacini	Cinnamomum zelanicum	"
Nagakesara	Mesua ferrea	"
Karpura	Cinnamomum camphora	"
Candana	Santalum album	"
Tila	Sesamum indicum	"
Bamsalocana	Bambusa arundinacia	"
Tagara	Valeriana wallichii	"
Avala	Phyllanthus emblica	"
Talisapatra	Abies webbiana	"
Pippali	Piper longum	"
Haritaki	Terminalia chebula	"
Sthul jiraka	Nigella sativa	"
Citraka	Plumbago zelanica	"
Sunthi	Zingiber officinale	"
Vidanga	Embelia ribes	"
Marica	Piper nigrum	"
Bhanga	Cannabis indica	20
Sugar	-	40

Dose— 1 *tola* (approximately 12gms), the dose of *Cannabis* comes to 3gms per day.

In his article *Indian Herbal Remedies*, Khare (2004) further discusses the dose by part of plant used, utilizing 125-250 mg of powdered leaf as a classical preparation for healing.

Classical preparations included:

- ❖ *Dhanvantari Nighantu*--- where *bhangaa* was administered as an intoxicant, digestive stimulant, diuretic, expectorant and aphrodisiac.
- ❖ *Bhaavaprakaasha*--- a prescription drug for diarrhea, dysentery and insomnia.
- ❖ *Vrindamaadhava, Bangasena*--- internally and externally for skin disorders.
- ❖ *Yoga Tantra*--- vaginal pessaries using *bhangaa* as an ingredient to contract the vagina.
- ❖ *Folk medicine*--- where the juice and paste of leaves were applied to affected areas of scalp and skin to remove dandruff and vermin. Powdered leaves were dusted over wounds to increase the granulation action for healing. Poultices were also placed on local inflammations associated with neuralgia and hemorrhoids.
- ❖ *Madan Modaka and Kameshwar Modaka*--- both were sweet prescriptions to relieve sexual debility.
- ❖ *Jaatiphalaadi Churna/Bhaishajya Ratnaavali*--- was used in the treatment of dysentery and colic.

In the *Handbook of Ayurvedic Herbal Medicines and Formulae (2003)* we read about an Ayurvedic branch which spiritually deals with the treatment of mental and psychological diseases (psychic, somatic and psychosomatic) called the *Bhutavaidya*. It mentions 6 forms in which *Cannabis* was processed to create therapeutic formulations for these kinds of psychological conditions:

1. *Curna* (powder)
2. *Modaka* (round bolus)
3. *Vatika* (tablets)
4. *Leha and Paka* (linctus)
5. *Dugdhapaka* (boiled with milk)
6. Kvatha (decoction)

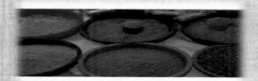

Ayurvedic preparations consisted of 51 main formulations made with *Cannabis*. These were a combination of herbs, vegetables, metals, animals and minerals which were standard inclusions in the practice of Ayurvedic medicine. They included:

13 *Curna* (powders)
24 *Rasa and vati* (Tablets)
11 *Modaka* (Round bollus forms)
3 *Avaleha and Paka* (Linctus)

Recommendations were made for these formulas to be drank with milk or ghee, accessing both the fat and water soluble properties of *Cannabis* (Touw, 1981). Other *Cannabis* preparations were mixed with food or combined in meals, chewed raw within *Piper betel* (Betel leaf) or smoked in a pipe known as *cilam*. Syrups made with finely ground *Cannabis* dried leaves were a sweet way of ingesting the herbal medicine. This was a classic homemade preparation and recommendation, that only the terribly determined to live an extremely long celebrant life would under... or should I say overtake.

IMMORTAL FORMULA
From the *Handbook of Ayurvedic Herbal Medicines and Formulae* (2003).
One liter of cow's milk mixed with one kilogram sugar and boiled together. When the mixture becomes thick syrup, 400gm of powdered *Cannabis* is added to 50gm each of 8 other medicinal herbs. Mix well. Let cool. Then add 500ml each of honey and ghee. Mix very well. Let the mixture stay within a heap of grain for a month reciting mantras daily, prior to use. Thereafter, a dose of 5gms daily is recommended for rejuvenation and well being. The accompanying recommendation is this, celibacy, and a diet of milk and rice only. This should be continued for a period of 300 years to avoid disease and aging.

PAINFUL PILE REMEDY (Touw, 1981)
Ingredients: *Bhang*, *Curcuma longa* (Turmeric), Onions, warm sesame seed oil.
Directions: Combine all the ingredients and apply externally to the affected area.

The above formulas were prepared with a variety of plant parts depending on specific indications. Often the female part was preferred when the physician intended to synergize and enhance the treatment, remember energetically the female part was considered bitter, thus potentiating assimilation in the digestive system.

Tibet
Momea, a Tibetan preparation possibly included human fat or lymph, of which I think quite interesting, honey, milk, butter and of course *Cannabis* (Touw, 1981).

Mediterranean
Nepenthe, a formulated drug in Homer's *Odyssey*, was a brew where the most active ingredient was *Cannabis*. Macerating the aerial parts in the recipe created the formulation ((Hamilton, 1852, Griffith, 1847).

United States
Fenner's Formulary provides a suppository formula containing *Cannabis*:
325 mgs lupuline (an alkaloid extracted from hops),
65 mgs *hyoscyamus* (Henbane) extract,
130 mgs monobromated camphor and
32.5 mgs *Cannabis indica*.

Cannabis was widely used to treat gonorrhea, particularly in homeopathy, in fact an 1839 homeopathic journal *American Provers' Union* mentions therapeutic formulas and uses for it (Hamilton, 1852).

Scudder (1898) formulated with *Cannabis* in two ways depending on the stages of gonorrhea. During the early stages of gonorrhea he combined *Cannabis* with *Veratrum* (Corn Lilies) or *Gelseminum* (Cranesbill) and with *Actea* (Black Cohosh) in the later stages of the disease.

China
Hua-T'o a famous "surgeon" made *Ma-fei-san* translated as the "bubbling-drug medicine" a concoction of 190-265 A.D to be used as an anesthesia during operations; the blend contains *Cannabis* (Touw, 1981).

Middle East and Far East
Majoon-e-Falaksair is a classical compound consisting of *Cannabis* as practiced in classical *Yunani Tibb*. A prescription for this formula was recommended for premature ejaculation and spermatorrhoea. It was/is made available over-the-counter (Khare, 2004). *Malack* a Turkish formula identical to *Majek* found in India consisted of nutmeg, cloves, camphor, and juiced *Cannabis* (Hamilton, 1852).

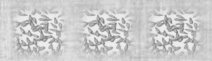

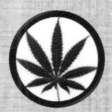

CAUTIONS AND ANTIDOTES

"I'll be the first to admit that herbal medicine is not risk free. To benefit from using herbs, you need to have some basic background information. Then you need to have confidence in the herbs you use and in any herbal practitioner you consult".

~The Green Pharmacy by James A. Duke, PhD

Around the globe ancient and eclectic physicians warned of the following in the overuse of *Cannabis*:

Contraindications and Cautions
Cannabis should never be used during pregnancy (Duckett, 1989).

China
Chinese claimed that *Cannabis* leaves may cause contact dermatitis, and the pollen, hay fever. They believed that

smoked herb may cause a loss of concentration, vomiting, and a heightened sense of pleasure (Naegele, 1980).

Europe
Hahnemann[35] claimed contrary to Middle Eastern physicians Ibn Sain and Yahya ibn Sarafyun; *Cannabis* causes exhausition (Hamilton, 1852).

South America
In South America, Duke J. A. (1986) asserts *Cannabis* leaves were substituted for tobacco in certain regions increasing cases of emphysema, cancer and heart disease.

Antidotes

Europe
Pliny the Elder[36] offered antidotes pepper and honey to toxic effects of *Cannabis* (Touw, 1981). In the

Flora Homeopathica (1852), it is written that reactions from large doses of *Cannabis* required sour lemonade and small doses of camphor.

---

[35] A German founder of homeopathic medicine of the 18th century.
[36] A Roman naturalist and philosopher of 23-79 A.D.

India

Indians had a longterm practice with *Cannabis* whether for spiritual, recreational or medicinal purposes. They witnessed many cases where the resin if taken in large quantities created insanity (Smith, 1883). In 700 B.C the *Susruta Samita* describes *Cannabis* root as a toxic substance when taken excessively (Handbook of Ayurvedic Herbal Medicines and Formulae, 2003). Because of their longterm relationship with *Cannabis*, Indians learned to use creative antidotes for its toxic effects. Generally, toxicity was avoided and therapeutic activity was gained by boiling it in cow's milk and/or frying it in cow's fat, *ghee*.

Also, to manage overdose Ayurvedic physicians administered these interesting antidotes according to the *Handbook of Ayurvedic Herbal Medicines and Formulae* (2003):

1. **Purgation**---suggesting the patient to ingest sour substances, then take a head bath with coldwater,
2. **Unction/Anointing**---by combining sandlewood paste, camphor and cold water and placing on the individuals head,
3. **Fragrants**---using cooling flowers,
4. **Sleeping**--- in cooling beds only,
5. **Use of cooling herbs**---a combination of *Piper betel* (Betel leaf), camphor and cloves,
6. **Garments**---wearing silk and fragrant garments,
7. **Drinks**---intake of a mixture of sugar, milk, ghee,
8. **Rest**---total bed rest was prescribed.

Overall, cooling, aromatic substances, cooling and soothing materials, and activities were highly recommended as antidotes to the narcotic effects of *Cannabis*. This makes sense with the exception of the female part, the plant was considered to have energetic properties described as hot, pungent and acrid!

 All societies conceded that *Cannabis* caused delirium (Neill & Smith, 1852) and broncihial dilation in healthy persons, laryngitis, apathy, psychic decline, sexual impotency with chronic use and failing genital function as well (Khare, 2004). Khare (2004) continues that certain constitutents like cannabinoids, increase heart frequency, peripheral vasodilation, systolic pressure while in the prone position and decrease while in the supine position. At this point I know *Cannabis* use for sexual function has caused confusion. One may want to apply an old wise phrase here... "everything in moderation." It seems the excessive dose or longterm use of *Cannabis* did an injustice but a little bit added medicinal benefits to the reproductive system specifically. Therefore validating Yunani Tibb observation of the plant as its initial effects or initial use is stimulating, and its final or longterm use causing an amotivational energy systemically.

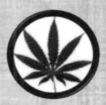

GLOBAL POLITICS: A SUMMARY

"The gods sent hemp through compassion for the human race, so that they may attain delight and lose fear...."

~Raja Valabba

In researching this book, I noticed over the years people have had a continuous love-hate affair with *Cannabis*. This kind of undulation created fear, confusion and misunderstanding of its use and its role in human health. These emotions are still current. The impact of politics has contributed to this paradigm, as political laws and actions affect societies as a whole. All societies who used *Cannabis*, show periods of consented use, ban, use and ban again creating a timeline that may resemble a *Cannabis* thread weaving in and out of society where a passionate tapestry depicts images showing like and dislike for the herb. China is an example of this where shamans were

condemned by ancient governments in *Cannabis* use, yet
revered the plant later for its fiber and food (Medical
Marijuana ProCon.org, 2006). Undeniably *Cannabis* in
industry, medicine, nourishment and recreation was
inevitable since its discovery which has led to undeniable
gross profits globally. On the contrary, people have taken
advantage of *Cannabis* and misused it as a quencher for
their thirst for control, greed, pleasure and power over
other peoples' social and spiritual life. This drive has
forced individuals to become detached from realizing their
natural role with the plant world. More profoundly, it has
distanced lives from understanding the self within the
natural order, which has lead to chaos and destruction on
a certain level. Political leaders have made decisions
according to the "trendy" relationship with *Cannabis*. This
has led to power and politics operating independent of the
beneficial impact of the herb. Political leaders have always
contributed to legal ins and outs of *Cannabis* in society
according to their economical or social interests.
Unknowingly or not, this affected people in both subtle
and monumental ways throughout *Cannabis* history.

Undoubtedly, there were times when political decisions
were made to deliberately discriminate and seclude
particular ethnic groups or classes who had grown to rely
on the plant like the Arabian working class during rule of
the Emir Soudon Sheikhouni from Joneima. In other
instances, political influences esteemed the plant,
encouraging farmers and physicians to use *Cannabis*
perhaps for economical profit. Today, *Cannabis* has

become a "confined" herb, only freely grown and taken by holders of permits and licenses. I am sure ancient practitioners, botanists, and agriculturalists would question this circumstance and that of any plant in this position. My explanation to the ancients would be something along these lines: we have delved deeper into an era of disconnectedness and irresponsibility, much which commenced during your time. Many leaders, not just political but health and social leaders have misled and divided us, causing us to lose trust in our fellow human beings and even in ourselves. Consequently, our relationship with nature and the planet, that is our home, has disintegrated into self-destructive patterns of behavior. Until we begin to re-establish our relationship with our true selves and our true home, we can never cultivate our relationship to the precious plants that share our ecosystem and nurture us, like *Cannabis*. As a writer of the *U.S Economist* March 28, 1992 bluntly stated, "Medicines often produce side effects. Sometimes they are physically unpleasant. *Cannabis* too has some discomforting side effects, but these are not physical they are political."

Let's review some of the political issues that have severed our relationship with *Cannabis* as medicine and that have served our societies as a whole....

North America
The following was summarized chronologically from the *History of Marijuana as Medicine 2737 B.C. to Present*, 2006, unless otherwise stated. One will notice that this chapter

covers U.S politics more than any other nation as it is the politics in the U.S that has created and influenced laws banning and unbanning *Cannabis* more than any other country in the world. In summary, U.S politics surrounding this plant is somewhat the global politics of it.

The year was **1619** when the first *marijuana* law was enacted at Jamestown Colony, Virginia "ordering" all farmers to grow Indian hemp seed. Consecutively, mandatory *hemp* cultivation laws were enacted in Massachusetts in **1631**, Connecticut **1632** and in the Chesapeake colonies mid **1700**. Its use was mainly promoted as a fiber rather than medicine. Then the **1850s** came and the US census recorded 8,237 *Cannabis* plantations of over 2,000 acres each! Ten years later, the Committee on *Cannabis indica* of the Ohio State Medical Society reported medical interest of *Cannabis* and its therapeutic use. Consequently in **1870**, the US Pharmacopoeia lists *Cannabis* as a medicine. **1856-1937** *Cannabis* began to hold a bad reputation as an intoxicant and lost its image as a medicine. Perhaps due to the following experience the reputation of *Cannabis* had began to decline: **1915** Utah passes the US state anti-marijuana law after Mormons who went to Mexico in **1910** returned smoking it. The Utah legislature enacted laws outlawing all Mormons smoking *Cannabis*, prohibiting it and any one found using it confronted with criminal law. Eventually, during this period, the states of Utah, California and Texas outlawed *Cannabis*. **1923** Canada adds *Cannabis* to its schedule of prohibited drugs called The Opium and Narcotic Drug Act. The states of Louisiana, Nevada, Oregon and Washington outlawed *Cannabis* in **1924** at The Second International Opiates Conference where it was declared a narcotic. **1927** the state of New York also outlaws *Cannabis*. The US government sponsors the Siler Commission to study the effects of off-duty smoking of *marijuana* by American servicemen in Panama, the report concludes *marijuana* is not a problem and recommends that no criminal penalties apply to its use. Then **1929**, the Southwest states in the US make *Cannabis* illegal as part of a move to oust Mexican immigrants, who were the majority of users in the country.

Enter **1933**; epitome of National *Marijuana* was at the the US Pharmacopoeia and Formulary. It was described as a narcotic poison, producing mild delirium as well as considered unstable and unreliable. Mid **1930s**, after the abolition of slavery, and after the Civil War, *hemp* declined in production as harvest and processing required intensive labor. By **1935-7** the US Treasury Department secretly drafted prohibitive tax laws called The Marijuana Tax Act of **1937** HR6385 (Snyder, 1971). The law called out for an occupational excise tax upon dealers and transferred tax upon dealings with *marijuana*; it was not yet totally banned but it ended the medicinal use of the plant in the United States, affecting its reputation throughout the world

(Snyder, 1971). Opposing this law, a legislative counsel of
the American Medical Association, Dr. William Woodward
testified the medicinal application of *Cannabis* especially
strong in psychotherapy treatment (Schaffer Library of
Drug Policy, 2006). Earlier Dr. John Bell had already made
claims to its useful intervention in mental illness. In **1937**,
the Hearst newspapers[37], published headlines and stories
insinuating Mexicans and *"marijuana* -crazed Negroes"
were "assaulting, raping and murdering whites."
Apparently these were false accusations, but influential
believers in congress parroted this claim. That same year,
President Hoovers Treasury Secretary, Mellon, who's
nephew in law, Harry J. Anslinger became the head of the
Federal Bureau of Narcotics and Dangerous Drugs
(FBNDD) in **1931**. In **1937** he was the ring leader assisting in
banning *Cannabis*, and branded the herb as the "worst evil
of all" (Bloomquist, 1971). As a result of his accusations, in
1941 *marijuana* was officially removed from the US
Pharmacopoeia. **1943** *US Military Surgeon* magazine stated
that *marijuana* was no more harmful than smoking
tobacco. **1957** a Wisconsin farmer harvested the last legal
commercial *hemp* crop in the United States.

[37] This newspaper supplied news across the United States from California
to New York in the 1930s to present.

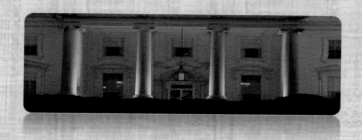

With the rise of hippies, the peak of African American social movements and numerous revolutionaries and activists, legalization movements for *Cannabis* began in the **1970s** and **1980s**. **1978** legislation permitted patients with specific disorders to use *marijuana* in 36 states (University of Washington, 2006). An upsetting, yet unsurprising entry found in the **1982** September edition of *Omni Magazine* stated that pharmaceutical companies like Eli Lilly, Abbott Labs, Pfizer, Smith, Kline & French amongst others produced man made drugs mimicking *Cannabis* such as Nabilone and Marinol or Dronabinol. However, these drugs were found to be less or ineffective in their treatment for the side effects from chemotherapy or AIDS symptoms for which they were prescribed. From this information these companies worried about losing millions of dollars US wide and billions to developing countries if *Cannabis* were legalized, so physicians continued to prescribe these pharmaceuticals. In **1988**, the administrative law judge declared that "*marijuana* in its natural form fulfilled the legal requirement of currently accepted medical use in the treatment of illness in the

United States" (University of Washington, 2006). Out of the push for its medical use, June **1991**, the Food and Drug Administration (FDA) was forced to institute *Cannabis* as a Compassionate Investigational New Drug (IND) for physicians who wished to prescribe to patients who had no alternative drugs for specific indications. It was then classified as a Schedule I drug.

United Kingdom
1928 the UK's Dangerous Drugs Act became law, making *Cannabis* illegal there.

India
1893-94 the government of India established a Hemp Commission which decreased *Cannabis* reputation in the medical profession and left it as an intoxicant.

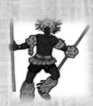

Africa
Cannabis was outlawed in Egypt during the 3rd century AD; its use was punishable by religious law and judicial authorities. To the Central West of Africa, the Bashilenge tribes[38] made *Cannabis* a part of jurisprudence (Spicer, 2002). Natives accused of crime such as adultery or thefts were required to smoke until they admitted their crime or lost consciousness. Further down South, Zulu and Sotho[39]

---

[38] A Central African Bantu people.
[39] These are two different South African ethnic groups.

young men smoked *dagga* prior to going to war, and won most of the wars. Its use is still well accepted in Africa (The Medical Museum: University of Iowa Health Care, 2006)

Jamaica

Ganjah smoking by Rastafarians was a symbol of protest against the Jamaican establishment and represented freedom from Jamaican laws (Spicer, 2002). The actions and cultural statements of Rastafarianism were extremely effective as they still are today.

Marijuana has journeyed around the world as an important commodity, a political member and a main character in

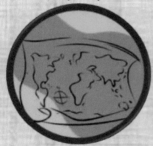 storytelling. It has served as a spiritual facilitator during Yogi tantric ceremonies, a mediator in African chieftain political deals, a remedy for Scudder's gonorrhea cases, and an object in Chinese dynastic attire. Adjacently, it has been a fugitive in Persia, Arabia and later Islamic movements, it has escaped into the hands of many like those in 14th century Ethiopian Orthodox Coptic churches and courageously into the backyards of underground American *marijuana* enthusiasts today. Throughout history the controversial fact remains whether in China, Greece, Persia, Egypt or America, it has been

92

associated with medicine in the act of healing, economic gains in the act of creating durable merchandise and in trading with distant worlds. We cannot ignore its value which unfortunately humans allow to propel crime games, an inevitable fact of anything illegal. Today, politics largely affects *Cannabis'* legal position in society. Yet we can make a difference by shifting our perspective towards it.

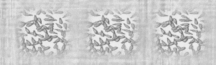

CONCLUSION: AFTER THOUGHTS...

I consider myself the voice of the plants, the gate keeper of the earth and the soul partner of nature. I defend her and all her Elements.
~Olatokunboh M. Obasi, MSc

Marijuana presents us with the opportunity to excel and connect ourselves with a greater purpose as well as the option of defeating ourselves in the distrust and excesses of the day. We have seen, fortunately, an undercurrent of global citizens who have begun to reclaim our rightful place as co-habitors of the planet. Through this undercurrent, I am hopeful that a global perspective of the plant emerges; one that fuses the lessons and gifts from the past; one that diverges our energy from politics back to plants. This text can serve as a guide to help us re-kindle that delicate relationship and ground ourselves with

the respect and love that once has a basis for our use of
the earth's great medicines.

Ancient physicians of systems like that of Ayurveda and
Yunani Tibb, used *Cannabis* for the benefit of suffering
humanity. What amazes me, still, is how contradictory the
association between spiritual wealth and criminal mischief,
marijuana has on our society. "*Marijuana* is symbolic of a
more passive, contemplative, and less competitive attitude
toward life than has been traditional in the United States.
It is usually denounced by people who like things the way
they are. Whether society accepts or rejects the drug will
undoubtedly have some influence on the evolution of our
national character" (Dell & Snyder, 1977; Snyder, 1971).

Thankfully, *Cannabis'* recent consideration for medicinal
use is only now becoming of interest, again. The plant has
always had medicinal potential. As a medical herbalist, I
have a wonderful appreciation for all plants especially
medicinal ones. I sympathize with this plant as I would a
person who has been a victim of abuse or one who has
been innocently accused of crimes not committed. Instead
marijuana has been finding ways to exist like you and me in
a world where people think they have control over
nature's magic. Right now *marijuana* is becoming popular
again because authorities are questioning its potential as
medicine after several years of unpopularity. During this
age of the Green Movement, *marijuana* offers us options
for sustainability of plants and the earth. Its growing
conditions do not have to be expensive due to its quick

maturity and versatile use of the whole plant. What may be difficult at this time as we try to place *marijuana* in a place of medicinal and commercial consideration, rather than illegal drug, is gaining realistic perspective of its role in society. Like all plants, medicinal or sustainable, we must see and approve of their potential as to how they benefit us and life on earth.

Let us evolve and recognize that we as people coexisting with other life forms on Earth must learn to accept the potential of all plants and be disciplined enough to limit our use of any single one. What I am alluding to is balance. In writing this text, I discovered that *marijuana* calls us to find balance and consideration. The balance must come in all realms of existence, time and space as we evolve spiritually, mentally and physically. *Marijuana* reminds us to learn to be considerate and accept of good things within Gaia, Pacha Mama, Dunia, Planet Earth or Earth Mother as they are.

Again, educating oneself with historical knowledge, present consciousness, and prospective information can assist in understanding, without judgment, this and any plant or life. This was the purpose of researching this book. To bring to you, the reader, historical knowledge of *Cannabis* that could influence your present consciousness to influence your future decisions around this plant. I hope I have fulfilled my purpose or at least contributed to the conversation.

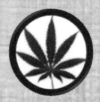

REFERENCE CHART

The chart below illustrates the concise historical association of *marijuana* and various countries already discussed in depth within the book.

Location	Medicinal Use	Preparation	Other Uses	Legal Status
Africa	Appetite stimulant, female disorders, uterine tonic, snake bite remedy, antiseptic, pain relief, antimicrobial, infertility, asthma, eye remedy	Both leaves and stems were prepared into tea, chewed, smoked	For jurisprudence by the Bashilenge tribe, used before wars by the Zulu and Sotho, baskets, currency, closing business deals	Pretty much legal

China	Absentmindedness, decrease heaviness in the body, beriberi, rheumatism, gout, constipation, female disorders, malaria, pain relief, eye inflammation, anesthetic	Flowering tops (unknown preparation), powdered, root paste, salve consisting of butter, oil and ground root	Clothing, shoes, sails, baskets, paper, ropes, fish nets, oil used for cooking, paints, vanishes and soap-making	Unspecified
India and South East Asia	Muscle relaxant, pain killer, sedative, fever reducer, sleep remedy, dysentery, sundry illnesses, appetite stimulant, quicken mind and speech, indigestion, aphrodisiac, anti-phlegmatic, hypnotic, nerve and urinary tonic, wasting diseases	*Bhang* drink: leaves and stems macerated in water, mixed with milk; *Ganja* sweets: flowering tops used in baked sweets; 1954 Indian Pharmacopeia official use as liquid extract from root and leaf	Commerce and trading, weddings and other festivals such as for Shiva followers, viewed as a sacred plant in Hinduism, enhanced concentration during prayer, Tantric sex	1893-94 categorized as an intoxicant substance by the medical community, ever since its value in medicine has diminished

Europe	Reduce childbirth pain, flatulence, earaches, edema, inflammation, antibiotic against gram-negative bacteria, anticonvulsive, painkiller, mental illness, immune tonic, gout, congestion, rheumatism, malaria, beriberi, burn treatment, ease menstrual pain	Root used for menstrual cramp painkiller, *Cannabis* green nuggets: *hashish*, sugar, orange juice, cinnamon, snail, cardamom, mocada nut, musk, pistachio, pinions; balm for childbirth	Gift at banquets for happiness and hilarity, used to make ropes and sails, smoked recreationally	1928 United Kingdom Dangerous Drug Act enforced law to illegalize marijuana
Persia and Middle East	Yunani Tibb qualifies its use for numerous ailments, reduce childbirth pains	As a beverage, Quannab (Cannabis seeds) burnt as incense and used for inhalation	Highly important trade item, cult activities for sedation of hashishin recruitees	Unspecified

America	Mania, whooping cough, asthma, chronic bronchitis, stimulant, tetanus, epilepsy, for alcohol withdrawal, colic, hepatitis, gonorrhea, sterility, impotency, tuberculosis, fevers, gastralgia, dysentery, cancer, painkiller, glaucoma, sciatica, infant diarrhea and teething, skin burns, bladder and prostate glands, urinary tonic, nerve tonic, excessive erections, pertussis, rheumatism, convulsions, hydrophobia, depression, female hyperesthesia in genitals	1842-1890 the most prescribed extract, Fenner's Suppository Formula including ½ grain of Cannabis	Divination, mystically, hallucinations, revelation of secrets, Rastafarianism as a politico-religious symbol, sacred smoke, for cosmic consciousness, smoked in groups as a symbol of trust and friendship, numbing those dying	**1619-1700** laws in Virginia, Massachusetts, Connecticut and Chesapeake colonies to grow hemp for industrial fiber use, **1870-** U.S Pharmacopeia list it as a medicine, **1915-** Utah passes US state anti marijuana law followed by California and Texas, **1924-**the second International Opiates Conference declared it narcotic, **1935-7-** U.S. Treasury Department prohibited tax laws on marijuana traders, **1941-** marijuana officially removed from U.S pharmacopeia **1978-**legislation permitted marijuana in 36 states, FDA instituted *Cannabis* IND

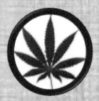

ABOUT THE AUTHOR...

*"You always carry within yourself the very thing that you need for the
fulfillment of your life purpose."*

~Malidoma Some

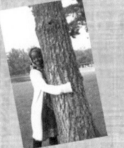

Olatokunboh M. Obasi is a
mother and medical herbalist
practitioner who graduated
from Tai Sophia Institute in
Laurel, Maryland with a
Master's of Science in Herbal Medicine. Raised in the Rift
Valley areas of Kenya and Tanzania, she has been a plant
lover for over 25 years. Her family now lives in South
Africa. She is the owner of Nourishing Botanicals LLC.
specializing in wellness care and Fair Traded Shea Butter
products. Her long term goal is to operate a successful
holistic global conscious center that serves individuals on a

community level to receive effective holistic health care as an option, offer spiritual guidance and beyond.

If you would like to connect with Olatokunboh M. Obasi you may contact her via her website at www.nourishingbotanicals.com or email her at nourishingbotanicals@gmail.com.

BIBLIOGRAPHY

Flora of North America. (2006). *Cannabis Sativa in Flora of North America.* Retrieved October 12, 2006 from http://www.eFloras.org.

Schaffer Library of Drug Policy. (2006). *Marijuana-History of the Intoxicant Use.* Retrieved October 3, 2006 from www.druglibrary.org/schaffer/Library/studies/nc/nc1b.htm.

Abel, E. L. (1980). *Marihuana: The First Twelve Thousand Years.*

Balick, M. J., & Cox, P. A. (1996). *Plants, People and Culture: The Science of Ethnobotany.* New York: Scientific American Library.

Bloomquist, E. R. (1971). *Marijuana: The Second Trip.*

Brown, O. P. (1872). *The Complete Herbalist or the People
Their Own Physicians by the Use of Nature's Remedies,
Describing the Great Curative Properties Found in the Herbal
Kingdom.* Jersey City: By the Author.

Cannabis Medicinal.com.ar. (2006). *History of Cannabis in
Black Africa and the Average Age .* Retrieved November 28,
2006 from
http://www.cannabismedicinal.com.ar/historyofcannabis/1
0.php.

Chaturvedi G.N, T. R. (1981). Medicinal Use of Opium and
Cannabis in Medieval India. *Indian Journal History Science* ,
31-35.

Dell, D. D., & Snyder, J. A. (1977). Marijuana: Pro and Con.
American Journal of Nursing , 630.

Duckett, R. (1989). *Basic Herbs for Health and Healing.*
Bronx: Sundial Product.

Duke, J. A. (1986). *Isthmian Ethnobotanical Dictionary.*
Gainesville: Scientific Publishers.

Duke, J. A., & Vasquez, R. (1994). *Amazonian
Ethnobotanicals Dictionary.* Boca Raton: CRC Press LLC.

Frank, M., & Rosenthal, E. (1978). Cannabis and Ancient
History. In R. Bud, *Marijuana Grower's Guide Deluxe Edition*

(pp. 3-13). Berkeley: Retrieved October 12, 2006 from
www.walnet.org/rosebud/ancienthistory.html.

Gray, R. J. (1894). *A Guide to the Study of Pharmacognosy or
the Essentials of Materia Medica of the Vegetable and
Animal Kingdoms for the Use of Junior and Senior Students
in the Buffalo College of Pharmacy.* Buffalo: Peter Paul Book
Co.

Griffith, E. R. (1847). *Medical botany, or descriptions of the
more importan plants used in medicine, with their history,
properties and mode of administration.* Philadelphia: Lea
and Blanchard.

Hamilton, E. (1852). *Flora Homeopathica.* London: H.
Baillere.

Handbook of Ayurvedic Herbal Medicines and Formulae.
(2003). Small Industry Research Institute, Indian Institute
of Consultants, Engineers India Research Institute.

Iverson, L. L. (2000). *The Science of Marijuana.* Oxford:
Oxford Univeristy Press.

Khare, C. (2004). *Indian Herbal Remedies.* New York:
Springer.

Kraemer, H. (1915). *Scientific and Applied Pharmacognosy,
Intended for the Use of Students in Pharmacy.* Philadelphia:
By the Author.

Levine, R. (2007). *Case Studies in Global Health Millions
Saved.* Boston: Jones and Bartlett Publishers.

Medical Marijuana ProCon.org. (2006). *History of Marijuana
as Medicine: 2737 B.C to Present.* Retrieved October 3, 2006
from http://www.medicalmarijuanaprocon.org.

Mikuriya, T. (1969). Marihuana in Medicine: Past Present
and Future. *California Medicine* , 110.

Moerman, D. E. (1986). *Medicinial Plants of Native America.*
East Lansing: Museum of Anthropology, University of
Michigan.

Naegele, T. A. (1980). *Edible and Medicinal Plants of the
Great Lakes.* Calumet: By the Author.

Neill, J. S., & Smith, F. G. (1852). *A Handbook of Materia
Medica and Therapeutics 2nd ed. rev.* Philadelphia:
Blanchard and Lea.

Nicoll, R. A., & Alger, B. E. (2004, December). The Brain's
Own Marijuana. *Scientific American* , pp. 68-75.

Raman, A. (2003). The Cannabis Plant: Botany, Cultivation
and Processing for Use. In D. T. Brown, *Cannabis: the genus
Cannabis* (pp. 29-47). Taylor and Francis e-Library.

Roodt, V. (1998). *Common Wild Flowers of the Okavango
Delta: Medicinal Uses and Nutrtional Value.* Gaborone: Shell
Oil Botswana (Pty) Ltd.

Scudder, J. M. (1898). *The American Eclectic Materia Medica
and Therapeutics 10th ed. rev.* Cinncinati: The Scudder
Brothers Company.

Small, E., & Cronquist, A. (1976). A Practical and Natural
Taxonomy for Cannabis. *Taxonomy* , 405-435.
Smith, J. (1883). *Domestic Botany: An Exposition of
Structure and Classification of Plants and of Their Uses for
Food, Clothing, Medicine, and Manufacturing Processes.*
London: MacMillan and Co.

Snyder, S. H. (1971). *Uses of Marijuana.* New York: Oxford
University Press.

Spicer, L. (2002). Historical and Cultural Uses of Cannabis
and the Canadian "Marijuana Clash". *The Senate Special
Committee On Illegal Drugs,* (pp. 1-32). Library of
Parliament: Retrived October 3, 2006 from
http://www.parl.gc.ca.

The dispensary of the USA, 25th Ed. (1955).

The Medical Museum: University of Iowa Health Care.
(2006). *Nature's Pharmacy: Ancient Knowledge, Modern
Medicine: Marijuana (Cannabis sativa)*. Retrieved October 5,
2006 from http://www.uihealthcare.com.

Touw, M. (1981). The Religious and Medicinal Uses of
Cannabis in China, India and Tibet. *Journal of Psycoactive
Drugs* .

United States Department of Agriculture Natural
Resources Conservation Service. (2006). *Plants Profile:
Cannabis sativa L. Marijuana*. Retrieved October 12, 2006
from http://plants.usda.gov/java/profile?symbol=CASA3.

University of Washington. (2006). *Medicinal Marijuana Use*.
Retrieved October 5, 2006 from
http://students.washington.edu/aed/archivemidget/2.htm.

Van Wyk, B.-E. G. (2000). *People's Plants: A Guide to Useful
Plants of Southern Africa*. Pretoria: Briza Publications.

van Wyk, B.-E., van Oudtshoorn, B., & Gericke, N. (2009).
Medicinal Plants of South Africa. Pretoria: Briza
Publications.

Information about the cover

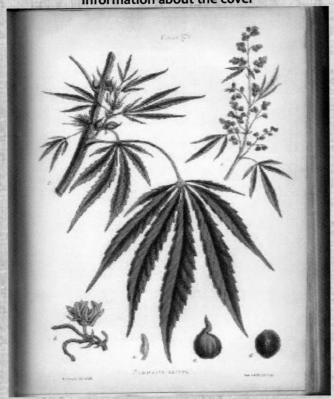

Cannabis sativa, Cannabis indica
(From 'Flora Homoeopathica', 1852 by Edward Hamilton,
illustration by H Sowerby)

CPSIA information can be obtained
at www.ICGtesting.com
Printed in the USA
LVIC06n2359161115
462920LV00011B/76